The Other Side of Impossible

The
Other Side
of
Impossible

---

*Ordinary People Who Faced
Daunting Medical Challenges
and Refused to Give Up*

Susannah
Meadows

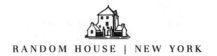

RANDOM HOUSE | NEW YORK

Published in the United States by Random House, an imprint and division of Penguin Random House LLC, New York.

RANDOM HOUSE and the HOUSE colophon are registered trademarks of Penguin Random House LLC.

This work is based on "The Boy with a Thorn in His Joints" by Susannah Meadows (*The New York Times Magazine*, February 1, 2013).

LIBRARY OF CONGRESS CATALOGING-IN-PUBLICATION DATA
Names: Meadows, Susannah, author.
Title: The other side of impossible / Susannah Meadows.
Description: New York : Random House, 2017. | Includes bibliographical references.
Identifiers: LCCN 2016044332 | ISBN 9780812996470 (hardback) |
ISBN 9780812986457 (ebook)
Subjects: LCSH: Medicine—Philosophy. | Alternative medicine—Philosophy. |
Mind and body. | BISAC: MEDICAL / Alternative Medicine. | HEALTH & FITNESS /
Alternative Therapies. | BODY, MIND & SPIRIT / Meditation.
Classification: LCC R723 .M353 2017 | DDC 610.1—dc23
LC record available at https://lccn.loc.gov/2016044332

Printed in the United States of America on acid-free paper

randomhousebooks.com

2 4 6 8 9 7 5 3 1

First Edition

Book design by Susan Turner

For Beau

If you bring forth what is within you,
what you bring forth will save you.

—The Gospel of Thomas

Contents

The Other Side of Impossible

1

Shepherd's Story, Part 1

The Leap

What if we'd never met Char?
—Darin and me

When my son Shepherd was three years old, he and his twin brother, Beau, took soccer lessons for the first time. They were so excited the night before their first practice that they slept in their uniforms—a purple T-shirt with a yellow star kicking the ball with one of its points. But when we got to the field the next day, Shepherd's enthusiasm evaporated. While Beau and the other kids zigzagged around the cones, Shepherd stood still and looked bewildered. When it was his turn to kick the ball, he seemed lost. After fifteen minutes, he walked off the field and sat down in my lap, saying he was too tired to play. We watched the other kids, and I pointed out to him the drills I thought he might enjoy, the ones that Beau was charging through. But Shepherd refused to go back to the field.

His reaction didn't concern me much—he was three, after all, and

I already thought of him, in the way that parents tend to categorize their children even as we tell ourselves we shouldn't, as not that interested in sports.

My husband, Darin, and I had recently noticed that Shepherd occasionally walked with a limp, but it was faint enough that sometimes when you looked for it, it was gone. Faint enough—though it seems incredible now—that we didn't connect it to his reluctance on the field.

I assumed that Shepherd would warm to his soccer lessons the next time around. He and Beau still donned their jerseys at bedtime and talked each night about "soccer school" at the dinner table. But the following Saturday, Shepherd broke into tears the moment he started to run.

That week we saw our pediatrician, who referred us to an orthopedist. When no injury showed up on the X-ray, the doctor said that arthritis was most likely the issue. Arthritis in a three-year-old? It sounded more odd than alarming at first, but over the next few weeks, as we waited to see the next specialist, we watched Shepherd spend more and more time on the couch. His stiff-legged walk became more pronounced, though he claimed that it was just an imitation. "I'm a penguin," he would say. Then he started having trouble getting out of bed.

A month after our first appointment, we went to see Dr. Philip Kahn, a pediatric rheumatologist at NYU Langone Medical Center, who gave Shepherd a diagnosis of juvenile idiopathic arthritis.

JIA is an autoimmune disease. It causes painful swelling in the joints. It can lead to stunted growth, disability, and, rarely, blindness.

When Dr. Kahn tested his joints, Shepherd denied that it hurt even as he teared up in pain. Our son was stoic, Dr. Kahn said, as the kids he treated often were. Shepherd turned out to have arthritis in both knees and both wrists, as well as in his left shoulder and elbow. Many months later a particular memory came back to me, its attendant mother's guilt harsh despite the passage of time: We'd bribed him to go to that last practice with the promise of ice cream.

Before driving home from the appointment, all four of us stopped for lunch at a hummus place that Dr. Kahn had recommended. We sat outside on the sidewalk, and Darin and I pretended that we were celebrating. This is great news, we told Shepherd. Now that we know what's wrong, you can take medicine that will make you feel better. Darin remembered thinking that we were lying to him, but he was trying to be more optimistic than he felt, for Shepherd's sake and for mine. Shepherd barely ate his lunch.

When we got home, I called my sister, Rae. She already knew that overwhelmed feeling of getting a child's diagnosis; she'd been through it with her daughter, who had severe asthma and fourteen food allergies. Rae talked about how that moment when you receive a diagnosis like this, for your child, eclipses everything. She tried to reassure me that if an illness isn't life-threatening, the fear eventually dies down, and coping with it becomes routine. Her daughter was three, the same age as Shepherd.

Rae must have made a similar call to me when she first got the allergy news about her daughter a couple of years before, but I have no memory of it. I'm sure I was sympathetic. I knew that having a child with allergies was difficult and scary, of course. But it was only after we found out about Shepherd's JIA, maybe not that first day, but sometime in the weeks afterward, that I realized I'd really had no idea before about what she was dealing with as a mother. I called her and told her I was sorry. Partly because I hadn't fully understood it, even though I don't think I could have. I don't think anyone can. But I also wanted to tell her I was sorry for what she went through because I knew now how much there was to be sorry for.

That day of Shepherd's diagnosis, Rae mentioned that a friend of her sister-in-law, a woman named Char Walker (short for Charlotte), sent her son's arthritis into remission with alternative medicine. Did I want to talk to her? I told Rae that I didn't, that we liked Dr. Kahn and wanted to follow his advice for now. We were starting Shepherd on a course of naproxen, a relative of the nonsteroidal anti-inflammatory ibuprofen. We didn't want to mess around with something that might not work when conventional treatments were known to be effective.

What I thought that day but didn't say to Rae was, *We don't want to waste time talking to a kook.*

SHEPHERD'S ARTHRITIS SPREAD WHILE HE was taking the naproxen. Joints in his fingers ballooned, and he developed nodules on his knuckles, which were suggestive of serious rheumatic disease. He started wetting his pants more frequently because, we realized after too much time, his fingers hurt so much that he couldn't pull his pants down.

We went back to Dr. Kahn, who said it was time to confront the painful inflammation in Shepherd's joints with methotrexate, a commonly used treatment for juvenile idiopathic arthritis.

Inflammation is supposed to be our friend. The heat, swelling, redness, and pain we're all familiar with are usually signs that this important immune system function is doing its job of fighting off an infection or helping us recover from an injury. Many different immune cells take part in inflammation. Some induce pain, perhaps to force us to rest and heal. Others—our white blood cells—attack bacteria or other foreign matter directly by gobbling them up. Inflammation can be incredibly destructive—that's how it defends us from invaders so effectively. But sometimes our immune system goes haywire and starts striking innocent tissue. When inflammation is inappropriate in this way or doesn't know when to stop, it becomes *our* enemy.

This is autoimmune disease: immune cells fighting against oneself. Excessive inflammation can also increase our risk of cancer and is a factor in many other diseases including obesity, diabetes, and heart disease.

Methotrexate works by suppressing the immune system, which mistakenly attacks the joints of children with JIA. In significantly higher doses, methotrexate is used as chemotherapy. Even at the dose Shepherd would be getting, a minuscule fraction of that, methotrexate could still cause nausea, dizziness, and drowsiness. The list of more serious possible side effects was terrifying to me—including liver damage and increased risk of lymphoma—even though Dr. Kahn told us that those risks were practically nonexistent.

Shepherd had polyarticular JIA—meaning five or more joints were affected. Children with this kind of arthritis are unlikely ever to outgrow it; Shepherd would probably be on medication for life. What were the long-term effects of taking this drug on three-year-olds? This question tended to visit me in the middle of the night, when Dr. Kahn's reassurances that methotrexate was safe gave the least amount of comfort.

As my anxiety about the medication churned, I talked to my friend Andrea about it. She's a doctor. I knew what she would say, and I needed to hear it. She told me, "I don't think you have a choice." Somehow, as I suspected it would, hearing that the decision to give Shepherd methotrexate was out of my hands brought some relief. Though the effect was fleeting, for the time being at least, I couldn't worry about what I couldn't control.

The pills were orange, Shepherd's favorite color. When I first gave them to him, he was enthusiastic about taking them. The real coup: His twin brother, Beau, didn't get to have them. But watching my son gulp the pills down defeated me. It reinforced an image of Shepherd as sick, forever dependent on a drug I felt afraid of, however unreasonable his doctor might tell me that fear was.

But this was our only choice.

Unless it wasn't.

One morning, while the boys were at preschool and Darin was out of the house, I decided to call Char Walker. She answered the phone, and within minutes I was crying to this woman I had never met. It was my first experience with the healthcare underground, women and families supporting each other, offering possible leads and kindness when traditional medicine wasn't enough.

Char told me that when her son Shane was an infant, only a month old, he started waking up seven or eight times a night screaming and crying, which he continued to do for a year and a half. He didn't have any symptoms that she could see. What was wrong? Soon she was crying every night, too. And then, at around eighteen months, he learned to talk and told her what hurt: his leg, his hip, and his wrist. Once they had the diagnosis of JIA, Char realized her son had proba-bly been in pain every night of his life.

Char was a social worker and massage therapist who worked with cancer patients at NorthShore University HealthSystem outside Chi-cago. When Shane's rheumatologist presented methotrexate or steroid injections as the only options, Char was horrified.

Because she worked in the integrative medicine department, which combined Western medicine with complementary interven-tions developed outside the mainstream, she knew there were other things to try in order to combat inflammation. And she wanted to try them first.

Char told me that Shane's rheumatologist disapproved of her deci-sion to delay drug therapy. Char said, "It was like, 'What the hell are you doing, lady?'" She remembered the doctor telling her, "I don't think it's going to work. I've been doing this a long time." Char said the doctor warned her that she risked stunting her son's growth and dam-aging his joints, not to mention prolonging his pain. (Shane's rheuma-tologist declined to speak to me on the record, though she had Char's permission to do so.)

Char dug into medical literature databases. From a naturopath she learned about an anti-inflammatory Chinese concoction called four marvels powder, which is made from two roots, a seed, and the bark from a decorative tree. Naturopathic medicine combines healing practices developed hundreds of years ago with more modern primary care. Emphasizing stress reduction, nutrition, and herbal supplements, among other interventions, the idea is to optimize the health of the body as a bulwark against disease.

Char also sought guidance from her colleague Dr. Leslie Men-doza Temple, the medical director of NorthShore's integrative medi-cine program. Dr. Mendoza Temple had experience with treating inflammatory arthritis. Char had come up with an extensive diet and supplement regimen. While wary of the risks, Dr. Mendoza Temple was comfortable giving the program a three-month trial. "I tried everything that I knew was safe to see what would work," Char told me.

I grabbed my pen and paper and started taking notes. No gluten, the protein in wheat, barley, and rye. No dairy. No refined sugar. No nightshades—a group of plants that includes potatoes and tomatoes— which are thought by some to be pro-inflammatory, as is sugar. Every day, Shane took a probiotic, those supplements of bacteria that are either the same or similar to the microorganisms found naturally in the body. Plus two tablespoons of sour Montmorency cherry juice and at least 2,000 milligrams of omega-3 fatty acids from fish oil, for their anti-inflammatory properties. Instead of naproxen, Shane took a combination of ibuprofen and Tylenol to lower his overall intake of nonsteroidal anti-inflammatories, which can be hard on the gut. And a quarter teaspoon, daily, of the Chinese herbal medicine called four marvels powder.

Char said she believed that her son's arthritis was caused by something I had never heard of before—leaky gut syndrome, a concept that had been accepted in alternative circles for years despite a name that asks you not to take it seriously. Leaky gut is based on the idea that inflammation in the gut damages the intestinal walls. As a result, the normally tight junctions between the cells that make up the intestinal wall's lining loosen. Then, like a careless bouncer, the barrier starts letting through undesirables, various proteins or bacteria that would normally be turned away. Once they've breached the wall, the hypothesis goes, these materials make their way into the surrounding tissues where they don't belong. These uninvited guests set off the immune system, which mounts a defensive, inflammatory reaction to get rid of them. The problem is that, in this scenario, instigators keep coming through. So rather than wage a quick and dirty fight that limits destruction, the inflammation is dragged into a sustained, drawn-out war.

What could have caused the inflammation in Shane's gut in the first place? Char suspected her son had an allergy or sensitivity to dairy and gluten, common perpetrators. She also implicated antibiotics because they can decimate protective, good bacteria, along with the bad. A week before Shane started waking up so frequently, he had been given antibiotics for a 104-degree fever. By the time he was one, he would have at least five more courses of antibiotics for urinary tract infections.

After Char told me this, I remembered that my son Shepherd had started limping not long after taking amoxicillin for pneumonia. There was no proof of causation, of course, and lots of children take antibiotics and don't get arthritis, but it was a detail that added to my big stack of nervous realizations.

Six weeks into the alternative therapy Char had put together—the no sugar, no gluten, no dairy, no nightshades diet plus fish oil, probiotics, and Chinese herbs—Shane Walker started feeling better. After three months, his arthritis pain was gone. When I spoke to Char, Shane had been in remission for almost two years. This was much better than anything we were told we could expect—although it is true that Shane's chances of remission were also greater than Shepherd's. Shane had three joints affected, whereas Shepherd had sixteen, that is, polyarticular.

A week later, we told Dr. Kahn about Shane Walker's story and floated the possibility of following the same course. Dr. Kahn wasn't familiar with leaky gut but agreed that it wouldn't be harmful to try Char's regimen in addition to the medication Shepherd was already taking. There was one part of it he was opposed to, though. Shepherd hadn't grown in at least four months so Dr. Kahn didn't want us to cut gluten-containing grains and dairy out of his diet—two major categories of food. We understood his point, but we were determined to give the complete protocol a shot. We weren't going to feed Shepherd less, we explained; we would make substitutions.

Dr. Kahn was adamant that, whatever we did, we not take Shepherd off the methotrexate. In fact, he wanted to up the dose from 10 milligrams to 15, because we were seeing the full effects of the initial prescribed amount and Shepherd was still in pain. He now woke up sobbing in the middle of the night, saying his ankle hurt. And arthritis had leached into his toes.

We agreed to stay on the methotrexate while we pursued Char's protocol.

Dr. Kahn jotted down "four marvels powder" in Shepherd's chart with a good-natured smile. He once told us about a patient of his whose Chinese grandmother was giving him, along with his medication, a tea that appeared to be helping. He was a believer, he'd said, in anything that worked.

I was nervous about keeping Shepherd on methotrexate, but Darin didn't share my squeamishness. He had always been more comfortable with pharmaceuticals, more trusting in general. I had to admit that Char's protocol was iffy. I was desperate to find a way to solve Shepherd's problems without the drugs; maybe my hope was misplaced. What if Darin was right and methotrexate was the only effective course? Darin worried that I might start insisting on no medication at all, and that I'd win.

Taking Chinese herbal medicines, of course, isn't without risk because they contain pharmacological compounds like any drug—and have pharmacological effects. "We forget that numerous medications we use may be extracted from plants before going through chemical manipulation or purification," says Dr. Leena Mathew, an anesthesiologist and specialist in pain management at NewYork-Presbyterian Hospital/Columbia University Medical Center.

One significant difference between an herbal remedy like four marvels powder and a pharmaceutical, says Dr. Mathew, is that the Chinese herbal medicine's side effects aren't well understood. As I later learned, one of the chemicals in the mixture *is* known to be harmful to pregnant women and infants. Still, four marvels has been used for over a thousand years to combat inflammation.

Other kinds of supplements—vitamins, minerals, botanical materials, and the live microorganisms of probiotics—aren't necessarily safe, either. It's an unregulated industry. The law doesn't require manufacturers to prove that their supplements work or even that they won't hurt you. Some of these products have done real harm, as Dr. Paul Offit, chief of the division of infectious diseases at the Children's Hospital of Philadelphia, writes in *Do You Believe in Magic?* And some contents have turned out to be different from what was on the label.

In the case of herbs from China, certain supplements have been found to contain toxic heavy metals. Through the hospital where she worked, Char bought four marvels powder that had been subjected to third-party testing. She was kind enough to be our supplier.

The omega-3 fatty acid supplements Shepherd took are generally safe, but they can extend bleeding time, according to the National Institutes of Health's National Center for Complementary and Integrative Health, the federal government's lead agency for scientific research on complementary medicine, treatments outside of Western medicine used in conjunction with it. (Alternative medicine, as the name suggests, refers to nontraditional therapies used in place of conventional medicine.)

Probiotics, another item on Char's list, have a good safety record, according to NCCIH, although there have been some reports linking them to serious infection in people with underlying health problems. As for knowing what you're getting, some supplements carry the stamp of the U.S. Pharmacopeial Convention, or USP, which does third-party verification.

I wasn't concerned that Shepherd would become malnourished from cutting out gluten-containing grains and dairy. He ate a range of vegetables, fruits, nuts, seeds, healthy fats, and proteins, in addition to other grains, such as whole oats. "No one food is ever essential," says Marion Nestle, a professor of nutrition, food studies, and public health at New York University. "Eating a variety of the others should work just fine." This seemed to be the case for Shepherd. "Humans evolved to be omnivorous. The wider the variety of real foods in the diet, the more it is likely to provide essential nutrients," Nestle says. But the more restrictions there are, the greater the risk that the body won't get what it needs.

At the time that we adopted Char's protocol, a lot of my attention was focused on trying to make substitutions for some of the things Shepherd loved to eat that contained gluten and dairy. As parents of allergic children know, shopping for and cooking special meals, and supplying special snacks to be kept in Shepherd's own special bin in the classroom, and making sure he had a special treat for when other kids had birthday parties and took in cupcakes he couldn't eat, is a huge job. I'm not sure I could have managed it if I hadn't been working only part-time, especially with all of Shepherd's appointments. It's an example of how having financial resources—in our case, we made up for my lost income by continuing to live in a small space—made these kinds of extracurricular efforts doable.

Although we eventually found the dairy-free mozzarella that melted reasonably realistically, the gluten-free bread that seemed less brittle than others, and the unsweetened nut milk that tasted the best, I ended up feeling like I had to make most things myself. For example, when I couldn't find a cereal that hit all of my marks—gluten-free, dairy-free, not-processed, no sugar—I started making my own granola. I burned and swore my way through most batches.

I did take some satisfaction in my more successful alimentary ventures. Sunday night had always been pizza night in our family. It became dairy-free-mozzarella-and-sausage-on-corn-tortilla night, and it was no less the rage with Shepherd and Beau. This was following several failed trials with weird gluten-free dough creations, including one that you poured into a pan.

Of all the specialty products we cycled through, it was the pancake mixes for the dietarily restricted that were the least disheartening. You could find brands that weren't filled with junk and that produced a product with surprising verisimilitude to the real thing. They also had a shocking ability to maintain their essential pancakeness even when I shoved spinach, collard greens, or other vegetables in them. I admit that I'm proud that my children came to think of pancakes as green. They became such a staple—for breakfast or dinner—that when Shepherd was asked to take a food into his classroom that was traditional in his family, he took in pancakes. And that plate of verdant, tapioca flour, coconut milk offerings went—I kid you not—like hot cakes.

CHAR SAID IT HAD TAKEN six weeks for Shane to start feeling better. Dr. Kahn and Darin agreed that it would be okay to hold off on increasing the methotrexate until we gave the diet and supplement experiment that much time.

But at the five-week point, on Char's regimen and the same dose of methotrexate, Shepherd seemed to be getting worse. He was nauseated and could barely eat for the two days after taking his weekly pills. If I could talk him into going to the playground, I'd have to carry him home. Beau pointed out that he was stronger than his brother, who'd always been his equal.

Shepherd now spent entire afternoons on my lap. I usually made a point of asking Beau if he wanted to sit there, too, so he wouldn't feel left out. They each got one of my legs, but that didn't stop them from skirmishing over turf. I remember having to tell them again and again that there was room for two. And I remember feeling pinned down and frustrated, eyeing all the things that needed to be done, unable to get to them.

Shepherd, who was now almost four, started using a stroller again, and we went to a physical therapy, occupational therapy, or doctor's appointment almost daily. I told Beau he could go to a friend's house or stay home with a babysitter, but he asked to go with his twin. "I want to keep Shepherd company," he said. While Beau had always been sweet, we also knew he was being affected and shaped by Shepherd's condition, too. He was becoming overly dutiful, as if by kindness he might fix the situation himself, or at the very least not add to our troubles. None of us were unscathed.

And then there was Shepherd. I was afraid that being sick was how he thought of himself. That worry was often crowded out by a worse one: What if nothing worked, not even a higher dose of medication?

Conversations between Darin and me became pain diaries. I would report on everything that hurt Shepherd that day, whether I'd accidentally brushed against his swollen fingers and made him cry. We no longer slept, and we moved through our days in a fog of depression. Our initial gratitude that at least Shepherd didn't have a life-threatening illness lost its power to console us. We believed that our lives would always be less happy.

Darin and I never went out. If we made plans, we always broke them. We just kind of closed up shop. But I couldn't quite keep out my friend Phoebe. She called me every day. She didn't miss one. I don't think she asked how Shepherd was doing or how I was. She just called. To this day, I tear up whenever I think about her doing that.

WE DECIDED TO GET A second opinion from Dr. Lisa Imundo, who at the time was the director of pediatric rheumatology at NewYork-Presbyterian/Columbia University Medical Center.

Dr. Imundo wanted to more than double Shepherd's dose of methotrexate. I asked her about the potential connection between eating certain foods and inflammation. She had treated thousands of kids with arthritis, she said, and diet changes did not work. I tried to explain leaky gut, but I'm sure I was stammering and blushing. She handed me a piece of paper with a list of hospital resources that included a name next to the words "complementary medicine": Elena Ladas. I could continue the conversation with her.

After Dr. Imundo's drubbing of Char's regimen, Darin was in a froth. A top doctor in New York just said Char's plan wouldn't work, so it must be true. In general, Darin is almost pathologically easygoing. Now he was cornering me in the kitchen to press his case. "Shepherd is in bad shape, you are in bad shape, I am in bad shape," he said. "What the hell are we doing?" I promised that I would agree to up the dose of methotrexate immediately after the six-week deadline, if he would give it until then.

Darin says now that I was steely and shut down, and he remembers worrying that this was the kind of thing that broke up marriages, that if Shepherd didn't get better, he didn't know what would happen to us.

That month, I lost my purse, then my suitcase, and then I got into a car accident. Though it wasn't serious, the boys were in the backseat. I called Darin and cried. "I can't handle it. I can't handle it. I can't handle it." He brought home a pink orchid that night. I made an appointment with a therapist.

A couple of days shy of six weeks, with Shepherd still struggling, I heard back from the complementary-medicine researcher whose name Dr. Imundo had given me. Elena Ladas's message was simple and direct. Yes, she said of Char's regimen, she'd seen that kind of approach work before. She even threw in a recommendation of her own, an anti-inflammatory supplement called Zyflamend.

Maybe we weren't fools after all, I thought.

That short phone call from Elena Ladas was the thing that pushed us to the finish line.

At six weeks—to the day, right as the deadline came due—Shepherd woke up and, for the first time in months, got out of bed himself. I'd gone into his room to help, as I did every morning, and found him standing in his pajamas. "Mommy," he said, "my knees don't hurt anymore." He was probably wearing the pajamas with the skateboarding monkeys. Beau was probably groggy, still lying in the bed adjacent to Shepherd's. Honestly, I really don't know. When I think of it, there's only Shepherd, standing there, not crying. I was too stunned to say anything before he scampered out to the kitchen for breakfast.

Within several months, all of his arthritis pain was gone. It seemed to pass out of his body joint by joint, exiting his toes and knees first and then onward up his body, as if he were stepping deeper and deeper into curative water.

After Shepherd held steady for months, we started weaning him off the methotrexate. Dr. Kahn was keen to get Shepherd off the medication, too. At one point during the process, after we'd taken the dosage down 25 percent, Shepherd had a little flare-up. Dr. Kahn considered raising the amount of medication again. I asked if we could give it a bit of time to see if Shepherd's body settled down on its own. It did, and Dr. Kahn told me something that was really nice to hear, for what it said about him as much as me: "Good mom's instinct."

We kept going, and Shepherd was eventually weaned off the methotrexate entirely. The boy we thought of as "the old Shepherd" came back, the goofball with a cloud-breaking smile that activates his one dimple. He initiated running races—and wasn't always the most gracious when he won. He improvised what he thought was karate. He pirouetted. While Shepherd was sick, Beau had shot past him in height. After the arthritis faded, Shepherd grew taller than his twin, and he started to close the gap in weight. While his immune system was suppressed by the medication, he got sick twice as often as Beau. That side effect went away, too.

Over the next year, Shepherd had five flare-ups. Two of them were on the heels of taking antibiotics for an infection. The other three came after he accidentally ate gluten. He had a chocolate-chip cookie, a couple of bites of toast, less than a quarter of a sandwich on sourdough. Each time, he felt pain within twenty-four hours, and it lasted as long as two weeks.

To be clear: There is no proof that it was Char Walker's diet and supplement regimen that drove away Shepherd's arthritis, or her own son's. Shane's case may be more striking because he didn't take methotrexate. But a study of two, of course, is not a study at all.

Spontaneous remission is one possible explanation. Even though Shepherd was on medication and a restricted diet, maybe neither of those interventions was responsible for his recovery. Maybe the arthritis vanished on its own for reasons we don't understand. It has happened to children with JIA, Dr. Kahn told me.

All the same, methotrexate works for many children, and its effects can kick in later than the expected four-to-six-week window. But, again, children like Shepherd, with polyarticular JIA, aren't expected to be able to come off medication. We tried so many things at once for Shepherd that there's no way to know for sure what worked or what combination of things had an effect. But even Dr. Kahn told me he believed the dietary regimen may have contributed to Shepherd's recovery. "I'm mystified by children on a daily basis," he said. "I've seen kids paralyzed, unbelievably critically ill. I don't know why they get better. The main thing is, if a kid's better, run with the football, you know? I'm thrilled."

WHEN SHEPHERD TURNED SEVEN, ALMOST four years after we began to try complementary therapies by ourselves, he was still without pain and off of medication. He ate a diet that included a wide range of whole foods. But he still avoided gluten and dairy. So there was more to do for Shepherd. But what?

Even so, we knew that we'd gotten incredibly lucky with his health. Darin didn't call it prayer, exactly, but he told me he made a point of thinking about how grateful he was every day.

Though it had been years since Shepherd's recovery, I don't think I ever looked at him without scrutinizing how he was moving. I realized that that would probably always be the case, but every time I looked I never saw anything but a gleeful little boy.

2

Instead of an Introduction

A Community of the Defiant

AFTER SHEPHERD RECOVERED, I WENT LOOKING FOR AN EXPLA-nation. I discovered that I wasn't the only one who'd searched in the wilds of unfinished science. It turns out that there is a whole community of us, people who are pursuing unfamiliar ways of healing, determined to solve the unsolvable.

The people I met found themselves in that same border town across the line from Proof, just as isolated and unsure as we had been, and yet unwilling to turn back. What struck me most about them was their extraordinary talent for hope.

And also perseverance. They are remarkable in particular ways that helped them push through the marsh of medicine, and of everyone else's skepticism, to seek help and answers when there didn't seem to be any. Many of them found purpose in the quest itself. "There's

meaning and beauty in all of it. Illness is negative and scary and difficult, but it's an opportunity for change and growth," says one, Annie
Salafsky, a farmer in Washington State. "It's a call to arms completely."

The people whose stories I tell in this book, all women, didn't do
it by themselves. They had what it took to find their own way, but they
had support from their families and from various health practitioners,
too. One of these helpers has an extraordinary story of her own, also
included here, of how she developed a therapy—despite lacking a
medical background—that already seems to have helped many children.

All of the people I write about are uncommonly confident and
independent. Hardheaded, even. They show how effective a vital ego
can be. They made me wonder about a connection between a forceful
attitude and survival, or success, how certain qualities, beliefs, and
experiences might enable us to dare to make a run at the unheard-of.

So I reached out to scientists who are researching agency and
stick-to-it-iveness, and how our minds affect our bodies. I looked into
why some people may be more resilient than others—how our instinct
for survival can be shaped and reinforced, and how helplessness can
be learned. I explored the advantages of having a gritty, determined
personality. I also found out about the discovery of brain circuitry that
may explain why some of us have hope. It could be that the resolve
embodied by the people in this book didn't just help draw them into
the unknown; it may even have boosted the climb back to health.

Science has long acknowledged that how we think influences our
recovery. That's why placebos are factored into experiments—to es-
tablish what part of a drug's positive effect results from the belief that
you're going to get better by taking it. And yet, in certain medical en-
vironments it's still not considered okay to say there's a link between
how we think and how we feel. "We have only recently begun to en-
tertain the possibility that our minds also contribute in a fundamental
way to health and vitality," says Dr. Jeffrey Rediger, a psychiatrist on
the faculty of Harvard Medical School and the medical director for
the Harvard-affiliated hospital McLean SouthEast. He tells me about
intriguing results of some small but rigorous studies looking at cancer

patients. Dr. Rediger says that "the will to survive, the strength and purpose to one's commitment to health, seemed to be one of the central pieces in why some people recovered or lived a lot longer than we think they should have."

I am someone who believes in science, who believes in vaccinating my children, who believes in—and depends on—the care of good doctors. I am reporting here on interventions that lack scientific proof because, in a way, this is a book about not knowing—and persisting anyway. It's about reaching the point when experimenting seems to be the only thing left to do. It's about people who just don't give up. These are also human stories about the effect that trial and error has on families—the conflicts, the confusion, the personal strain, the fear, and also the hope.

The people in this book constitute a small, unscientific sample of fighters. Rather than being prescriptive, their stories are about the fact that families are doing this, are pressing on, and achieving surprising results.

On a frontier, there are no firm answers, but I went anyway, as a parent first, and then as a journalist. Now I'm reporting back.

Most of the people here never fully left the medical establishment. What they share is a frustration that most doctors will understand all too well: There's simply not enough science available to guide some of us, and some of our children, toward healing. We need answers now, and we are not willing to wait.

3

Shepherd's Story, Part 2

The Science of Our Guts

INCREASED INTESTINAL PERMEABILITY AND INFLAMMATION

ONE THING WE DO KNOW ABOUT OUR BODIES IS THAT THERE IS A link between the gut and inflammation, and we've known it for some time. Dr. Kahn told us, during our visits—and amid his serious talks with Shepherd about Batman: If he can't fly, why does he have a cape?—about a colleague, Dr. Jose Scher, who was researching how the gut and inflammation worked together.

I called Dr. Scher, the director of the Arthritis Clinic at the NYU Hospital for Joint Diseases—and he rattled off four different kinds of arthritis that are connected to inflammatory responses in the gut. One kind is linked to celiac disease, a gluten intolerance. Dr. Scher told me he'd also seen some of his autoimmune arthritis patients improve by removing gluten from their diet.

Early on, a celiac blood test had come back negative for Shepherd, but could he still have a sensitivity to gluten, something short of full-on celiac, that triggers a similar inflammatory response? A small 2006 study published in the journal *Gut* (you probably subscribe) points to a possible yes. The researchers found significantly elevated antibodies—proteins produced by the immune system to attack invaders—in the digestive tracts of rheumatoid arthritis sufferers but not in their blood. (Rheumatoid arthritis is not JIA, but the two are related.) The antibodies were targeting various foods. So not only were many of the arthritis patients found to have some level of intolerance to certain foods, but the issue wouldn't necessarily have been detected by a blood test.

Leaky gut, meanwhile, turns out not to be conjecture after all. "A lot of doctors and people may think that leaky gut itself is sort of a froufrou alternative concept," says Dr. Sanford Newmark, a clinical professor of pediatrics at the University of California, San Francisco, and the medical director of the clinic at the UCSF Osher Center for Integrative Medicine. "The real name is 'increased intestinal permeability,' and it is a definitive, scientific fact."

Leaky gut's embrace by alternative medicine followers seems to have tainted its reputation, like a rock star whose image suffers if his fans aren't cool.

Alternative remedies have a reputation of their own, for making claims of efficacy in the absence of evidence; also for causing adverse effects in some cases. Chiropractic manipulations have torn arteries, acupuncture needles have led to serious infections and punctured organs, and high doses of some vitamins have been found to increase the risk of cancer, as Dr. Paul Offit writes in *Do You Believe in Magic?*

While leaky gut is real, there's no proof that it causes autoimmune conditions, including JIA, by allowing the wrong proteins and bacteria through the intestinal wall. But some scientists see hints that one leads to the other. For one thing, having a leaky gut is a common denominator in many autoimmune diseases.

One big clue came in 2000 when Dr. Alessio Fasano, the director of the Center for Celiac Research and Treatment at Massachusetts General Hospital and a gastroenterologist, figured out how gut permeability could be modulated. He and his team of researchers discovered that when a particular human protein was released, the normally tight junctures in the intestinal wall opened. The protein, which the scientists named zonulin, acted like a key to the gates in a medieval city's fortifications.

There's a good reason for having this system: The ability to change the permeability of our intestinal wall protects us from unwanted bacteria.

Here's how it works. We evolved to keep bacteria out of the small intestine because if they settle there, they steal our food. Dr. Fasano, who is also a visiting professor of pediatrics at Harvard Medical School, explains: "We reached an arrangement with bacteria: You can stay here in my body, but you have to be all the way at the end in the colon. By then, I've digested what I can digest. So the leftovers that I cannot use, you can use." He's referring to dietary fiber, which our bacteria seem to crave. "In exchange for hosting you," Dr. Fasano says, resuming his conversation with bacteria, "you give me something from this feeding that will be beneficial for me." (More on what we get out of the deal later.)

Despite this understanding with bacteria—here's dinner if you stay in the large intestine—we still developed a wealth of defenses, such as stomach acid and bile, to kill bacteria off in case they venture into our small intestine or stomach and steal precious morsels that we'd otherwise benefit from. But, if some plucky bacteria survive this acid and bile thrashing, "we have one last chance to get rid of these folks," says Dr. Fasano; that is, releasing the protein zonulin in order to increase the space between the cells of the intestinal lining. Then, water can flow into the small intestine and wash the bacteria out from where it doesn't belong. "Like when you go to the bathroom and flush the toilet," says Dr. Fasano. This same chain of events protects us from harmful infections. Our zonulin lets water into our gut to rinse the invaders out of us, otherwise known as diarrhea.

It's an effective setup when it runs properly. But there's a potential glitch. It turns out that gluten can activate the release of zonulin.

So, to use another analogy, if zonulin is the button on the elevator that holds the doors open, gluten is the little kid who can get carried away with pressing it; zonulin can increase the permeability of the intestinal walls even when there's no enemy afoot. For most people, gluten's shenanigans aren't a problem, says Dr. Fasano. The openings in the gut lining squeeze shut soon enough.

In a certain percentage of us, though, the doors in the intestinal wall get held open for too long. This is how we wind up with security breaches: Materials, including bacteria, that would normally be refused entry for size are allowed to get past our defenses and into our tissues where they have no business being. The immune system may then perceive these foreigners as the enemy and attack them with exaggerated inflammation. This is what we talk about when we talk about leaky gut.

I have to ask Dr. Fasano something that I've been wanting to ask for a long time: *What is gluten's problem?* "This goes against my business because I live with demonizing gluten here," Dr. Fasano says of Mass General's Center for Celiac Research and Treatment. "I think it's a big misconception to make this the evil of the twenty-first century. Our ancestors spent ninety-five percent of the time on the procurement of food. What agriculture did, i.e., wheat, allowed us to unleash the creativity to build the Coliseum or to invent the phone so you and I can have this conversation." Dr. Fasano, who, it must be said, is Italian-born, digresses into the many uses of wheat, the most prominent of the gluten-containing grains. "You can do pasta, you can do pizza, you can make beer. . . ."

Okay, but it's also clearly no angel for some of us. And it turns out, gluten *is* unique. There's a reason it's always in the police lineup: Gluten is the one kind of protein our body can't fully digest, Dr. Fasano says.

He explains that we don't have the enzymes to be able to break gluten down all the way. Its tight bonds are what we love about it— they give bread its elasticity. But the protein's recalcitrance seems to be the reason it can cause problems. Its distinctive chunkiness seems to be read by our bodies as harmful bacteria: Our immune system's response to gluten, including the release of zonulin, is the same as its response to a suspected pathogen—any microorganism that makes us sick. Our body treats gluten like an adversary that needs to be attacked and flushed out.

So it's a case of mistaken identity. "It was not meant for gluten to do that"—to register as an enemy, says Dr. Fasano. The whole thing is a fluke.

For what it's worth, Dr. Fasano eats gluten, but in moderation. "Diversifying nutrition is a must. If I eat two pizzas a day, I will get sick, no question about that."

I reached out to the Grain Foods Foundation, an advocacy group, to see if anyone there wanted to stick up for the oddball protein, but a spokesperson declined to comment.

Since discovering the mechanism behind leaky gut, Dr. Fasano's group has assembled more evidence that a hyper-permeable gut lining is potentially related to autoimmunity. They've shown in an animal model of type 1 diabetes that if you stop gut permeability by inhibiting the release of zonulin—so the intestinal wall gates stay shut—the animals don't get the disease. In a clinical trial of the same drug that stops zonulin, people with celiac disease who were exposed to gluten were protected from symptoms. "So leaky gut is clearly part of the story," says Dr. Fasano, who owns stock options in the company that developed the zonulin inhibitor.

As the drug makes its way through clinical trials, anticipation is growing. It's often mentioned in gastroenterology journals as a potential therapy for celiac disease patients, one that would allow them to eat gluten-containing grains.

This had me thinking, too, of Shepherd.

Veena Taneja, a researcher and associate professor of immunology at the Mayo Clinic in Rochester, Minnesota, also sees compelling signs of a cause-and-effect relationship between a leaky gut and autoimmunity. The arthritic mice she works with in her lab often have hyper-permeable gut linings. She and her team have also compared the bacteria in healthy individuals with rheumatoid arthritis patients and have identified bacteria that are overgrown in the RA group. "When we tested one of those bacteria in arthritic mice, which have human genes, it increased gut permeability," she tells me.

Another telling observation from Taneja's lab: Some of these same suspect bacteria resemble a particular kind of human protein, so when the immune system tries to get rid of the invaders, it may accidentally go after its own cells. Arthritic mice given these bacteria were found to have an increase in antibodies to self-proteins. The body attacking itself is, of course, the very definition of autoimmunity. In fact, the human protein that resembles the bacteria is a major component of cartilage—found in our joints—and is considered a target of inflammation in people with rheumatoid arthritis, says Taneja.

OUR MICROBIOME

Many researchers are less focused on the stealthy bacteria of a leaky gut than on the entire community of microorganisms that live in and on our bodies. These microorganisms are referred to collectively as the microbiota or microbiome. They consist primarily of bacteria but also include fungi and viruses.

Their numbers alone suggest how significant these microbes are. We are made up of approximately thirty trillion human cells. The total number of microbes in us is roughly the same amount, according to a 2016 report in *PLoS Biology*.

We are only half ourselves.

This population of bacteria as a whole seems to play a major role in whether we develop disease or not.

"Traditionally we've thought about disease as being caused by a specific bacteria," says Julie Segre, a senior investigator at the National Institutes of Health's National Human Genome Research Institute. But now scientists think it is more about the *balance* of a bacterial community. "It may be that if you have disease-associated bacteria within a healthy population, then the other members of the community may keep that 'bad' bacteria in check."

And if you throw off the delicate ratios in the gut's microbial community, the bad actors might get too much leeway.

An example of how this works is *Clostridium difficile,* or *C. diff,* a bacterial infection that causes severe diarrhea. People don't get sick from acquiring the bacteria; it's already in the guts of some healthy individuals, kept in line by other bacteria. It's only when something like a course of antibiotics wipes out the peacekeepers that *C. diff* can turn pathogenic.

In fact, having an unbalanced bacteria population, or dysbiosis, is associated with a variety of diseases including autism, multiple sclerosis, irritable bowel syndrome, celiac disease, allergies, asthma, cardiovascular disease, obesity, and rheumatoid arthritis. As Mass General's Dr. Fasano puts it with his usual flair, "It's not a good scene when some bossy microorganism takes over."

Throwing off the balance between good and bad bacteria could lead to a hyper-permeable gut lining because the immune system responds to elevated numbers of bad bacteria by sending in pro-inflammatory cells to wipe them out. And too many pro-inflammatory cells—too much inflammation—can cause collateral damage.

Scientists still haven't completely figured out the mechanism, says Mayo Clinic's Veena Taneja, but she says that excessive inflammation can indeed harm the gut lining. "If the integrity of the gut lining is gone, that is when contents of the lumen"—intestine—"go out of the gut." This could explain how having an inflammatory response in the gut from a food intolerance could lead to trouble.

I ASK DR. FASANO WHAT he makes of Shepherd's story. He's not the least bit surprised to hear that Shepherd recovered from arthritis after he cut out gluten. "We see stuff like this often," Dr. Fasano tells me. After years of getting skeptical looks about the course we followed, I'm a little bit stunned to hear this.

He explains what he thinks happened. "In your son, possibly, again, this is wild hypothesis, he had this problem because genetically he was predisposed, because let's say he had an infection—"

He did, I say. Plus he took antibiotics. "Here we go," Dr. Fasano says.

In a 2015 study in *Pediatrics,* a leading medical journal for pediatricians, taking antibiotics was associated with an increased risk of developing juvenile idiopathic arthritis, even after factoring out the infections the children were being treated for. Dosage and timing mattered. The more antibiotics given, the higher the risk of disease, and the link was strongest within a year of diagnosis. What makes this study especially convincing is its scale: The medical records of more than 450,000 children in the UK between the ages of one and fifteen were analyzed. The results are meaningful because an estimated one-quarter of the antibiotics prescribed for children—and approximately half of those prescribed for acute respiratory infections—may be unnecessary, the authors write.

Dr. Fasano explains how the antibiotics Shepherd took may have affected him. "That changed the microbiome, increased gut permeability and so on and so forth. Once you have increased permeability, even something subtle that in general doesn't do too much harm, i.e., gluten, now causes a problem," he says. In other words, it holds the doors in the intestinal wall open for too long.

"This loss of barrier function, therefore, will increase antigen trafficking all the time!" says Dr. Fasano, antigens being all those things that incite an immune response, including undesirable bacteria and proteins—even gluten, the door-holder, itself—that ease through the gates in the intestinal wall that would normally be closed to them. When you stop eating gluten, he says, the wall can get back to working again like it's supposed to, shutting out inappropriate materials. As a result, the JIA gets under control.

This makes me wonder: If Dr. Fasano knows that this is possible, why don't more doctors? Why aren't the rheumatologists and gastroenterologists talking to each other? And why did I only first hear about how gluten might affect arthritis from a mom in suburban Chicago?

It reminds me of when I was chatting one afternoon with another mom while our children had a playdate. It was right after Shepherd had recovered and I told her about it. She said, "So how do you control his arthritis? With diet?" She was so nonchalant about it, as if everyone knew where the pot of gold was. I said to her, "Now, how do you know about that when our doctors don't?" She's a physical therapist. She told me she'd heard about it from her patients.

But even knowing what he knows, Dr. Fasano says he would not tell all children with inflammatory arthritis to stop eating gluten. I ask him, Why not? Because there is probably only a small percentage of kids who would get better, he says. As with many diseases, there are likely different ways of making the wrong turn to JIA, he says. If you take all kids off gluten, he estimates that maybe 10, 15, or 20 percent of them will get better. "Ideally we will find those who will benefit and put them on a gluten-free diet, so something that can be beneficial will not be vilified by the criticism of: How can you claim that this diet is beneficial when only a small percentage of people will benefit from it?"

I tell him that that's the difference between the two of us. I say, "As a mom, I think, 'If it's not going to do any harm, and we don't have a biomarker yet, let's try.'"

He comes right back at me. He says, "Let me tell you." And then he does: "I made the statement to a journalist"—me—"who writes for a reputable newspaper about what is scientifically correct," he says. "As a father, if I have a kid with autism or JIA and I read that [a no-gluten diet] is beneficial, with all due respect, who gives a boop—I will go for it. What am I going to lose? There are no side effects. It's not that I'm putting my kid in a hyperbolic chamber. Or that I'm going to put him on harmful drugs that can give really bad side effects. You want me to wait for you to find the biomarkers blah blah blah? Well maybe it's too little too late at that point."

THE TWO GENOMES INSIDE US

While scientists continue to sort out the details of what exactly goes on in our guts, this much is already clear: We need a plentiful, diverse population of bacteria to be able to function properly as humans. Just how fundamental are our microorganisms?

Dr. Fasano points out that humans have about 25,000 genes. Kind of pathetic when you consider that worms have more than three times that amount. Wheat, which contains gluten, has over 150,000 genes! How is it, then, that—despite our comparatively lame numbers of genes—we're more sophisticated than a loaf of rye? The answer is that we are the sum of two genomes.

The first one is the human genome we're all familiar with, our set of DNA, that instruction manual for building and sustaining the organisms that we are. The second genome is the combined genetic material of the bacteria we house in our bodies.

It turns out that these two genomes—ours and our bacteria's—are in cahoots, sending chemical messages to one another, running together the show that is each of us.

So while our bacteria do the important but more menial jobs of keeping the thugs of the gut in line, as well as helping us digest tough carbohydrates in fiber and producing vitamins for us, they operate on a more sophisticated level, too. This second genome belonging to our bacteria trains our immune system to know how to respond when we're under attack, and, crucially, not to overdo it with sustained inflammation, as Justin and Erica Sonnenburg, married microbiome researchers at Stanford, write in their book, *The Good Gut.*

We—our human cells and our microbes/bacteria—are like close neighbors whose kids are growing up together, with the older ones telling the younger guys how to be cool. A lot older—bacteria have been around since approximately the beginning of time.

The first three years of life are the crucial period for this symbiotic relationship between the human and bacterial genomes, as the Sonnenburgs write. But if we don't do right by our bacteria—if we're exposed to infections and take a lot of antibiotics and don't eat enough fiber—we can wind up with a belligerent bacteria population. The right lessons won't be shared. Our bacteria will train our immune system to be hyperactive so that we unleash the weaponry—the destructive munitions of inflammation—even when it's not needed, leading to autoimmune disease. Studies have not established that antibiotics lead to the development of autoimmunity, but there is evidence that our microbiota can protect us against autoimmune disease.

The implications go well beyond autoimmunity. "What research has shown over the past decade is how the bacteria in our gut are wired into virtually all aspects of our health," Erica Sonnenburg tells me. "They are [not only] setting the dial on our immune system, determining the strength and pace of our immune responses to things like viruses, [but] they are connected to our metabolism, helping our body decide whether to burn or store extra calories, and more recently they have been linked with our body's central nervous system, potentially influencing our moods and behaviors," she says. "In so many ways these bacteria are redefining the way biomedical researchers view the human body, no longer as a single entity but as a composite organism or a walking ecosystem made up of human cells and bacterial cells."

A healthy microbiome is such a central player in our bodies that it's "a true organ," says Dr. Alexander Khoruts, a gastroenterologist and an associate professor of medicine at the University of Minnesota Medical School. "The microbiome has major metabolic functions. It's second only to the liver in its output of chemicals in our body. It talks to the entire body. It talks to the brain," says Dr. Khoruts.

We all have genes that put us at risk for various diseases. Whether we get sick or not depends on whether those genes get expressed. "The microbiome seems to be one of the most influential pieces of environmental pressure for our genes to change and therefore switch from potential problems to actual situations," says Dr. Fasano—in other words, the thing that turns on the disease or not. "We talk about autoimmune diseases," he says, "but you can extrapolate to cancer or to neurodegenerative diseases like Alzheimer's and so on."

DESPITE THE EMERGING SCIENCE THAT could possibly explain Shepherd's recovery from arthritis, we still couldn't know for sure what helped him. (For an in-depth look at the evidence for the omega-3s and probiotics we gave Shepherd, see the appendix.) At home, though, we believed that it was Char's diet and supplement regimen that did the trick. We marveled at how lucky we'd gotten that my sister knew someone who knew Char. And that she happened to be kind enough to help us. A busy mother of three with a demanding job, she spent time she didn't have on the phone with us and answering our emails. And mailing us four marvels powder!

This is one of the reasons I wanted to write about Shepherd, which I first did in *The New York Times Magazine.* Not everyone had a Char, so I thought I should share what may have helped Shepherd.

Darin and I still say to each other, *What if we'd never met Char?*

4

Terry Wahls

How Far Can Moxie Take You?

Courage is knowing you're licked and doing it anyway.
—Zach Wahls

DR. TERRY WAHLS EARNED A BLACK BELT IN TAE KWON DO WHEN she was twenty-three. When she was forty-eight, she had to start using a tilt recline wheelchair. She'd been diagnosed with multiple sclerosis, a disease that can disrupt the brain's ability to communicate with muscles.

As a result of the MS, Terry's muscles had atrophied from disuse. The athletic woman whose physicality had once been central to her identity now no longer had enough core strength to keep from flopping forward.

But industrious and independent, she'd never been one to go along with anything imposed upon her. She'd always flown her own flag.

Terry had grown up a misfit in the northeast corner of Iowa, on a farm near a town called Elkader. Every morning she woke up to the alarm bell of her father's call, and she and her two brothers would shuffle out to the barn to milk the cows or tend to the hogs before school. They made their way in the dark, except in summer when the sun's glow would just be starting to eke out from the horizon, as if through a tear in the ground-sky seam. At that hour the light was a weakling, but it would be enough to help them on their way. The children resumed their chores as soon as they got home from school.

Starting when she was eight, Terry would bring the cows in from the pasture, her forehead just peeking over their backs. In the distance, she could see the wind manhandle the tall grass. Invisible as it was, it made its airy presence known by moving what it touched, like a ghost carrying a candelabra.

There weren't birthday parties or sleepovers with other kids. There was so little money that replacing a broken light fixture in the kitchen was a strain. The kids each got one present on Christmas, a wallet, maybe, or a pair of overalls. One year, when the kids were little, Terry's brother Rick remembers his father smashing a syrup pitcher against a kitchen wall. They'd just lost a number of their hogs to a respiratory disease. He said some angry words about life being unfair. It wasn't until much later that Rick realized what had probably set his father off. It was the fact that they were eating pancakes for dinner because that was all they could afford.

Their father, John, had always been emotionally distant. Though their mother, Lois, was sparing with hugs, she was a more nurturing force. But when Terry was nine, both of her parents drifted out of reach. That year, Lois gave birth to a baby girl named Maryellen who had a heart defect and died within days.

The kids retreated to their corners. Terry wasn't great at reading social cues, and she'd always been happiest being alone. She spent time hanging out with her horses. She went through a foraging phase, walking her family's land to find wild asparagus, onions, or sorrel. She was never invited to parties but she can't remember now if she was even aware that they were going on. By high school she was well on her way to being six feet tall.

When she was sixteen, she started dating a boy from a neighboring farm, but that didn't offer the reprieve it might have. By then, she had figured out that she liked girls, but if anyone was on to her she never knew. Like most small towns in the '50s and '60s, Elkader was a place where no one talked about being gay. There were more churches than restaurants. There were no traffic lights in the county. There still aren't. There were sock hops in the basement of the Elkader Opera House. The bakery on Main Street was closed on Sunday so folks who wanted a doughnut after church would stop in on Saturday nights to stock up. A socially awkward lesbian was never going to fit in here. Terry remembers thinking as a teenager, "If the world could see what's in my head, they would not be very happy with me."

As a kid she was content—or at least resigned—to being on the outside. She was comfortable there. And because she'd never been a citizen of normal, she didn't have to abide by its laws. "For whatever reason," she tells me, "I've never felt obligated to do what people told me to do. I made my own decisions about what it was that was the right thing to do."

Which is why, when her father asked her to sign over the title to a cow her grandfather had given her to an entity called John Wahls and Sons, she said no. He needed ownership to be able to sell its calves. She said she'd be happy to do it if the name was John Wahls and Family. Her father started yelling. "That's not how it's done!" He grabbed the directory, opened it to a random page, and showed her how every other farm was named after the men and the boys. "See? This is how everyone else does it." To Terry this was not a persuasive argument. She held firm and kept her cow. She was ten years old.

Without a script she was willing to follow, Terry proved to be a natural improviser. When she was fourteen, she was especially close to one of her horses, a brown and white Appaloosa named Paladin. He'd follow her on walks around their property, scaring up pheasants. He would nudge her shoulder. She'd usually respond by scratching his neck and tickling his chin. But if she didn't give him enough attention, he'd nip her. It hurt, those chompers chomping her shoulder. She got a little tired of it. So the next time he did it, she turned and bit his nostril, drawing blood. Paladin never nipped her again. They remained friends.

Terry finally broke up with the farm boy, graduated from high school, and escaped to Drake University, where she majored in fine art. During her last two years she loaded up on science classes, too; by then she'd decided to pursue medicine. Her parents seemed confused by all of it, but her mother quickly became proud of her daughter, the doctor. Her father never gave her the impression he felt any delight. Years later, though, when she was invited to participate in her high school's distinguished-alumni parade, she overheard him telling the neighbors that he'd been the one to encourage her to become a doctor.

Terry's parents found out she was gay right after medical school, and it didn't sit well with them. Terry's mother didn't think homosexuals could be successful in life. By the time she moved to Marshfield, Wisconsin, to practice medicine, Terry was barely speaking to her father.

In her twenties, Terry went through a difficult breakup. Word must have somehow gotten back to her dad because one day he called to cheer her up. When she tries to tell me about what he said those decades ago, she can't get the words out. She takes a moment to fend off the tears and finally says, "He said, 'I know you're kind of gay.'" At first I think she's crying because the notion of being "kind of gay" seems kind of offensive. But it turns out she's crying because he'd finally acknowledged who she was. Even for someone as self-reliant as Terry, getting her dad's tacit approval meant something.

That basic need for parental acceptance notwithstanding, Terry was always uncannily sure of herself. When she was working in private practice in Marshfield in the '90s, she repeatedly ran for leadership positions and lost. One year, when she didn't get voted onto the executive committee, she wrote in her diary, "Still it is an old boys' network, and I am still an outsider and always will be." She kept at it—and kept losing. After yet another loss she wrote, "The phenomenon is sobering. The wall."

Around the same time, Terry started to be harassed by teenage boys in her neighborhood. "It seems," she wrote in her diary, "my neighborhood finally knows that I am a lesbian." They yelled something at her about "smelling the stench of a lesbian." She felt threatened but didn't consider leaving. "I view myself as tenacious and extraordinarily persistent," she wrote. "So time to prove that again." She went over to the house of one of the boys who'd taunted her and spoke to his dad. He agreed to rein in his son.

When Terry decided she wanted to have children on her own, she ran into that now-familiar wall. It was the tail end of the '80s, and as a single parent, she could not find a clinic that would perform in vitro fertilization. Sorry, one physician told her, but they didn't do illegitimate children. By that point, though, Terry was used to smacking up against red brick and equally accustomed to hurling a grappling hook up to the top. She eventually flew out to San Francisco, where a sperm bank was willing to work with her. "I am pioneering again," she wrote in her diary.

Her mother argued with her, warning that it would be too hard to be a single parent. Terry wasn't dissuaded. Once she was finally pregnant she wrote in her diary, "I tackled this alone. I face my fear of this alone and my triumph alone." At another point she scrawled, "Facing this alone. I will solve the problems." The entries reveal her already up-and-running resolve. They also show that like so many diarists before her, she leaned in to the drama of her life, embracing the challenges. It would be a crucial trait when MS hit.

Two days after her son, Zacharia, was born, Terry was excited to look up the birth announcement in the *Marshfield News-Herald*. When she flipped to the right section, though, she found no mention of her feat. She called the paper. When she was told it wasn't their policy to report a single-parent birth, Terry told the editor she'd be consulting with her lawyer. She hung up and realized she didn't have a lawyer. When she called the editor back, though, she was told to check the paper in two days. But, she wanted to know, have you made an exception for me or have you changed your policy? The editor said he'd have to get back to her. A half hour later he called back to say that from that point on they would be publishing birth announcements of all local children. When she went in for her postpartum appointment, the OB nursing assistant laughed and told Terry that the staff at the clinic had placed bets on how quickly she'd be able to get the paper's policy changed.

WHEN TERRY STARTED USING A wheelchair, it had been only three years since her MS diagnosis. The onset of the disease, though, was earlier; she'd had unexplained pain for years. Now her MS was progressing rapidly. She figured she'd soon be bedridden. At that point, she was a clinical professor at the University of Iowa Carver College of Medicine in Iowa City, teaching internal medicine to residents. She was also a staff physician at the Iowa City Veterans Affairs Health Care System, overseeing policy for her region. With her health in decline, it wasn't clear how much longer she'd be able to work. She realized that the cost of her care would end up burning through all of her family's savings. Her son, Zacharia, was twelve, and a second child, Zebediah, was nine. Terry also had a partner, Jackie Reger, who'd been a member of the family for seven years. The two would later marry.

As awful as Terry's fate seemed to her, she'd reached a certain level of acceptance and calm. "You get to a place," she says, "where you can finally just take every day as it comes."

But there was an aspect of her MS that still left her terrified. One of her recurring symptoms was acute facial pain. "The pain starts like an electrical jolt," she says. "It's so painful that I can't talk. I have this involuntary grimace. When it gets so severe, I can't maintain muscle tone to stand. The pain obliterates your ability to have controlled motor responses, controlled thoughts. All you have is this white noise of horrific pain."

As Terry's MS progressed, these episodes became more intense and more resistant to drug therapy—even three days of IV steroids was no longer enough to shut off the pain. It was also happening more frequently, as often as once a month. The fear that she could not figure out how to live with was: What if her face pain turned on and didn't turn off?

The answer she came to, which she never shared with Jackie or anyone else, was suicide. Once she recognized that there was this way out of her disease, she felt some relief. Not that the idea didn't also flood her with grief. But of the many things MS stole from her, the part she missed the most was a feeling of control over her own life.

Studies show, as we'll see later, that having a sense of control is a key factor in agency—in whether you take action or not. It is also a key factor in the stories of all the people in this book.

Terry was no good at taking orders, whether it was from an authority figure or her own failing body. Everyone would struggle to accept that change—it's a defining awfulness of any insurmountable disease. But for someone who'd always been in such command, the loss of power was especially tough to take.

She took some solace in resistance. It gave her a feeling of having a little control.

The idea of suicide was an off-ramp when Terry had been so sure before that there wasn't one. If she took it, it was at least her choice. She didn't focus on the actual act—she never did plan it out. Instead, she comforted herself with the fact that a second option existed. "You always have choices," she'd say to herself.

There was one hitch. It wasn't an option she'd ever want her children to choose. She was haunted by the prospect of being an example to them. Neither choice was tolerable, really: intractable pain for herself or, if she chose suicide, intractable pain for her family.

TERRY AND JACKIE'S LIFE TOGETHER had always centered on physical pursuits. Their first house, in central Wisconsin, backed up to a wide meadow. After a fresh snowfall, all four of them would descend on that blank, twenty-acre canvas to draw paths. The two women liked to put on skate skis and herringbone miles of state forest trails. As the days warmed, they swapped out their winter paraphernalia for bicycles, swimsuits, soccer balls, tents, and a canoe.

The first time Terry's kids saw her in a wheelchair, in 2003, it was disorienting and upsetting. Terry's daughter, Zebby, remembers her mom's performance the day the wheelchair was delivered. Terry attached a big smile to her face. "Look!" she said. "I'll be able to zoom around so much faster now. It's just for work because the VA is really big," Zebby, who's nineteen when I meet her, remembers her mom telling her. It was the truth. Terry was still able to use her legs. The fatigue that accompanied the disease was the more pressing issue. She'd gotten the electric wheelchair to help her make it to the end of the day.

Terry's daughter was just young enough at the time—nine years old—to feel reassured. "She said it was going to be okay so I believed her. Some of her invincibility remained," Zebby tells me. Zach, who was twelve, was more aware. Seeing the ramp in his mom's minivan jolted him. "It's here and it's not going away," he realized about her MS. "My mom's life as I understood it, as a parent and as an adult, was over. There was a finality about it," says Zach now.

Their mom had trouble sitting up at dinner. She would have to lean forward and brace herself against the table. It was hard to watch, and Zebby would pretend not to see it. "I felt like I was intruding on a very private moment, like when someone doesn't want you to see them cry," she says.

But it was difficult to be understanding all the time. On the scale of middle school mortification, being seen in public with your parents is traumatizing enough. Zebby suffered the additional embarrassment of being seen with a mother in a wheelchair. "I would go back inside and berate myself because it wasn't her fault," she remembers. "But it wouldn't change how I felt." Early on, Zach was resentful and angry. *Why do we have to deal with this? We're dealing with gay parents already,* he thought. "It was insult to injury," he tells me.

Terry kept up a front for her children. She'd done theater in high school and called on her old acting skills now. Zach and Zebby rarely heard her complain. But they also knew she was busy writing letters to them at night in case she got to the point of not being able to offer them guidance anymore. When I ask Zach what it was like in the house then, he has a one-word answer: "Quiet."

✿ ✿ ✿

MULTIPLE SCLEROSIS IS CONSIDERED BY most experts to be an auto-immune disease. It involves confused immune cells that attack the self rather than an invader. In MS, this inflammatory process damages myelin, the protective sheathing that covers nerve fibers in the central nervous system, as well as myelin-producing cells. Many people in the field believe that in addition to inflammation, there's a second process in MS that's more progressive and degenerative and leads to loss of both the myelin and neurons, according to Dr. Lael Stone, an MS specialist at the Cleveland Clinic. The disruption in the nerve pathways interferes with the brain's ability to tell the muscles what to do. When you try to send electricity through a damaged power cord, the lamp sits there dark, not knowing that it's supposed to be on.

The last several decades have brought the introduction of medications that can successfully slow the progression of MS. The most common form of the disease, called relapsing-remitting, is also the least debilitating and the most responsive to the available drug therapies. People with relapsing-remitting MS experience episodes of difficulty followed by recovery. The symptoms of tingling, numbness, balance problems, weakness, or even blindness can stick around for months before retreating. Drugs have been able to reduce the frequency of these exacerbations and may reduce disability. People with this type of MS often live normally for decades.

As time goes on, though, relapsing-remitting MS can develop into secondary-progressive MS where the trajectory is more of a downward slope. Another type of MS, primary-progressive, follows a similarly relentless path. Drugs tend not to be effective in both of these cases. Chemotherapy can sometimes level out the slide but can't be used for more than a couple of years.

In all forms of the disease, the fatigue that often accompanies it can be incapacitating, though some medications can help on this front. "The patients are furious with the medical community for inadequately addressing progressive MS," says Dr. Stone, the MS specialist at the Cleveland Clinic, who is also Terry's former neurologist.

When Terry was diagnosed in 2000, she turned to the medical literature to find out all she could about MS. The outlook, she learned, was even worse than she'd thought. She remembers reading that half of those diagnosed with MS had to quit working within ten years because of fatigue, and a third developed a gait disability, such as limping or stumbling. She found it too distressing to keep up her research on the subject. She knew she was getting the best care at the world-class Cleveland Clinic, which she commuted to. She would put her faith in her doctor. (The current outlook for newly diagnosed patients is slightly more encouraging. About half of those with the most common form of MS will experience difficulty walking fifteen years after onset.)

At the time of her diagnosis, Terry was still jogging, but she would soon have to give that up. Her neurologist, Dr. Stone, prescribed one medication after the next, including chemotherapy, but nothing could fend off Terry's worsening symptoms. The attacks of facial pain would knock out for days her ability to function.

Jackie was a nurse, so she was probably in a better position than most to be able to deal with Terry's degenerative condition—not because she knew how to take care of people, necessarily, but because she'd seen worse. She'd spent eight years working with cancer patients. "This didn't seem that bad," she tells me. "It wasn't fatal."

But there were also times, as there always are, when it was really hard on Jackie. Terry would want Jackie near her during bad flare-ups, so Jackie would lie very still beside her. But one move could make the facial pain go off again. It was exhausting, and Jackie would think, "Please fall asleep. Please fall asleep so I can get some rest."

As Terry's fatigue worsened, Jackie went with her to the medical device store in town. The two of them had gone in thinking it was time for something like an electric scooter that would help Terry conserve her energy. The owner of the store showed them the tilt recline wheelchair instead. "You might as well get this one," he told them. "Because you're not too far from it."

By that point, Terry's disease had likely transitioned to secondary-progressive MS. She could no longer expect periods of recovery and it was doubtful that any of the available medications would have a real impact. This new self, increasingly dependent on her family and now her wheelchair, was unrecognizable to her.

She'd put the medical literature away years before. But now that she was in a wheelchair, she got back to it. That future she'd been afraid to confront had started bleeding into her present; the jig was up. Perhaps by reading everything on MS, she'd find something her doctors had missed. A physician herself, she knew it was impossible to keep up with all the research, especially if you saw patients all day.

So every evening after saying good night to the kids and Jackie, Terry settled into her zero-gravity chair, which reclined so far back that it didn't exact any muscle use from its occupant. Then she would rev up her laptop. Even though she was used up by the effort it took just to get through the day, she would log on to PubMed, the mammoth database of biomedical literature maintained by the National Institutes of Health, scanning for all MS research. She would stay up for hours reading papers written in a technical language she scarcely understood. Since she was a clinician, not a researcher, her grasp of the ever-evolving scientific terminology and concepts wasn't all that firm. She kept having to stop to look things up.

At best, she hoped to slow the progression of her MS, even though chemotherapy had failed her—the only known option for people at her stage. Still she had to try. "Courage is knowing you're licked and doing it anyway," says Zach.

Terry seemed to have been primed her entire life to take on something as difficult as MS. "I wonder if knowing she was different from her family members (artist, lesbian) all her life has given her inner peace, happiness with herself, inner strength, locus of control," Jackie writes me in an email. "The ability to hear what others say but process it within oneself and make it real/true for you."

So when the disease started to overpower Terry, she refused to concede. The experts say there's nothing that can be done to stop her disease? Most people would take the word of professionals who've devoted their lives to treating and looking for a cure for MS. But when had she ever thought like most people? I mean, who bites a horse's nose?

It helped that she tended to be stubborn. "Stubborn, bullheaded, cantankerous," her brother Rick tells me. "She's smart and she knows she's smart," says her other brother, Denis. "It's always been the world according to Terry." Does that attitude perhaps signal insecurity? I ask him. "No," he says. "She's full of herself."

One of the things she hunted for online was information about clinical trials of experimental drugs that she might be able to enroll in. Then it dawned on her that even if she found a study that would take her, she'd have a hard time getting to it. (She'd started seeing a local neurologist because traveling to the Cleveland Clinic had become too difficult.) Next she tried to learn about drugs being prescribed off-label for MS—medications that were approved for different diseases that doctors thought might help other problems. But Terry couldn't figure out a way to search for studies of off-label uses.

She was running on hope fumes when she decided to venture from MS into research on other brain diseases.

She focused on animal model studies because they were the cutting edge. They were also the longest shot; if something worked in a rodent, the odds of those results being repeated in a human were minute. Terry knew that it could take decades for a discovery to make it through all the safety trials, let alone be incorporated into medical practice. She obviously didn't have that kind of time. She'd have to skip some steps.

THE MITOCHONDRIA FACTOR

After months of midnight digging, her shovel hit some interesting nuggets. A couple of papers mentioned that malfunctioning mitochondria could play a role in MS. Mitochondria are the tiny units within most of our cells that convert fuel into energy. They're often referred to as our cells' power plants but are involved in other functions as well.

Then Terry came across an article published in *Annals of Neurol-*

ogy titled "Bioenergetic approaches for neuroprotection in Parkinson's disease"—an unlikely attention grabber. The author, Dr. M. Flint Beal, wrote that there was considerable evidence suggesting that Parkinson's disease may be brought on, at least in part, by issues with the mitochondria. The problems included decreased activity along one section of the energy-making assembly line, as well as increased production of damaging toxins. The mitochondria in these patients were less efficient and more polluting, like old factory equipment. The article went on to describe certain nutrients such as creatine and coenzyme Q_{10} that had been shown, in animal models, to be effective at protecting the mitochondria and keeping them running optimally. In a ten-month study of eighty people with Parkinson's, Dr. Beal wrote, coenzyme Q_{10} slowed disease progression by 44 percent. A follow-up study, though, was less promising.

Okay, so Parkinson's wasn't MS, it wasn't even an autoimmune disease, but if mitochondria were a factor in both, then maybe the nutrients that had helped the Parkinson's mice would help her, too. She got out her calculator and set about translating the mouse-size doses of the protective nutrients to a human scale.

She started looking into what else was known about mitochondria upkeep. In one study, in *The Journals of Gerontology, Series A,* mice with an accelerated aging syndrome that were given a mixture of thirty-one specific nutrients lived longer lives. The list included garlic, green tea extracts, cod liver oil, and vitamins B_{12}, C, D, and E. This flood of good stuff, the authors suggested, protected against mitochondrial dysfunction, among other mechanisms of aging.

How might this have worked? When mitochondria produce energy, they also emit exhaust, little molecules known as free radicals. When too many of these collect in the cell, they can damage the mitochondria.

Antioxidants—hundreds of vitamins and other substances that are abundant in fruits and vegetables—are thought to mop up this toxic grime before it can cause trouble. Here was food again, offering a possible way to recovery.

MS is relatively rare, affecting an estimated 400,000 in the United States. But wearing out our mitochondria is thought to be a driving force in the decline that gets us all—aging.

Terry was well aware of how little bearing rodent studies had on sick humans because we're such different creatures. But if Terry was short on proof, she was now long on optimism. She'd thought she'd wrested back a little bit of control before, when she contemplated a way out of her facial pain. But this was a kind of control that wouldn't destroy them all. This was beating it.

Out came the calculator again. She spent hundreds of dollars at the local co-op on the supplements the mice got in both studies. She came home with B-complex vitamins, creatine, L-carnitine, lipoic acid, coenzyme Q_{10}, and others.

A note here on safety. Terry checked with her primary care doctor before taking the long list of supplements and got the go-ahead. But supplements still carry the risk that they might contain something other than what's on the label. And some, including the vitamin E that the long-in-the-tooth mice took, can increase cancer risk in high doses. As Dr. Paul Offit, author of *Do You Believe in Magic?*, tells me, "There are pretty solid data at this point that you can get too much of a good thing."

The risk is associated only with supplements, however. When we eat foods rich in antioxidants, we're physically prevented from overdoing it. "Your stomach is only so big for a reason," says Dr. Offit. And: "For people who eat diets rich in antioxidants, they appear to have less risk of heart disease and cancer."

Terry, who was unaware of any potential increase in cancer risk at the time, started downing fistfuls of pills every day. She can't remember now if E was included. After six months, she didn't notice any improvement and thought, "Hell, I'm wasting my money." So she quit.

The next morning she couldn't get out of bed.

On day two Jackie came in with her vitamins and said, "You better take these." Terry woke up the next day, got out of bed, and went to work. *Oh, this is really interesting,* she thought. A month later, she tried stopping and starting again and got the same result. She got support from her neurologist, Dr. Stone, who also reviewed the list of what Terry was taking.

While she was taking all those supplements, her fatigue and gait difficulties hadn't improved, but they hadn't gotten any worse, either. Terry wondered if the supplements were slowing down the rate of her decline.

She decided to self-experiment even more. Part of her role at the University of Iowa was to evaluate study proposals and help decide whether to give the research a green light. She requested that all applications having anything to do with brain function be funneled to her.

She came across one by a physical therapist proposing to use neuromuscular electrical stimulation on patients who were paralyzed from a spinal cord injury. The therapy had been used largely on patients with athletic injuries. An electrical current delivered to the muscle could cause it to contract and, as a result, could help prevent atrophy and even promote growth.

Terry got an idea. She called up her own physical therapist, David Reese, and asked if he would try electrical stimulation on her. Reese told her it was painful and exhausting therapy. Though he thought he could probably grow her muscles, he wasn't sure her brain would be able to communicate with them. All the same, he was up for trying. At that point, Terry was spending most of her time in her zero-gravity chair. She could manage ten minutes of exercise on a mat in the morning, but any more and she'd be too exhausted to go to work.

Reese attached electrodes to Terry's quads and back and turned up the charge. They needed enough juice to stimulate a visible contraction in the individual muscle. At the same time, Reese instructed her to try to do a volitional contraction herself. If the MS was impairing the communication between her brain and her muscles, Reese was trying to strengthen the signal.

After twenty-four minutes of absorbing electrical currents, Terry was flattened. "She came home wasted, just exhausted," says Zach, who'd picked her up from the appointment. But he remembers that she was smiling. "And she didn't smile very often at that point."

It was the best she'd felt in years. She was tired, for sure, but she also felt the euphoria that comes with a release of endorphins.

She acquired her own e-stim device so she could activate her muscles as frequently as possible. She did it at work, turning the dial down when she had to speak, in order to relax her grimace and get the words out. *If I'm going to fail,* she thought, *I want to have left nothing on the table.*

Terry spent all of her waking hours in intense, fizzing pain from the powerful electrical current; the machine was not approved to be operated this much at a time. She burned out a series of devices by overusing them. Zebby, who was then twelve, invented a superhero named Electro Lady. The character looked like a female incarnation of the Flash—with lightning-tipped eyebrows and a buxom bod. She even had an origin story; her powers were the result of an accident with her "electrostimulation thingy," Zebby wrote on the back of her sketch.

Meanwhile, the real Electro Lady wondered if her brain was getting all the nutrition it needed. She tunneled back into the literature and found an exhaustive, two-part report on dietary requirements for the brain in *The Journal of Nutrition, Health & Aging.* Dr. Jean-Marie Bourre, a member of France's National Academy of Medicine, wrote: "A number of findings show that dietary factors play major roles in determining whether the brain ages successfully or experiences neurodegenerative disorders." Omega-3 fatty acids, iodine, manganese, copper, and zinc, among others, were all relevant to either brain function or structure, he wrote. Terry's list of supplies for her brain grew longer.

In late 2007 it occurred to Terry that if she started eating nutrients in the form of whole foods, she might pick up hundreds if not thousands of beneficial ingredients science hadn't yet identified—or perhaps she'd find that these instruments worked better as a symphony.

She set off for the medical library on campus, but the collection on

nutrition was hardly robust. The librarians couldn't find any information connecting nutrients to their food sources. Terry turned to a different institution for help, "the University of Google," as she calls it.
The search engine came through with a menu, including liver and kelp,
among other temptations, she'd now be tucking into.

She'd been on the Paleo diet for five years, which excludes grains,
dairy, refined sugar, processed foods, and legumes, the plant family
that includes peanuts, beans, and peas. The diet emphasizes meats,
eggs, vegetables, and fruits—the kinds of things proponents say humans ate during the Paleolithic era. In fact, it was her former neurologist, Dr. Lael Stone, back at the Cleveland Clinic, who'd suggested
she look into it. Dr. Stone had come across the website of a Canadian
scientist named Ashton Embry whose son was said to have controlled
his MS for years by staying on the Paleo diet.

Dr. Stone tells me that for some time she has included diet and
exercise in the conversation she has with patients, in part because
many people with MS are also obese and have diabetes and high blood
pressure. The main reason, though, is that she's interested in anything
that might help her patients. "It's really hard to go through an entire
day of clinic and watch people you've known for ten, fifteen years
gradually get worse," she says. "We deal with an incurable disease that
we don't understand and every individual is different." So Dr. Stone is
constantly asking, "What else can we be doing?"

There's no question that some patients feel better when they try
certain diets, says Dr. Stone. No gluten, fast food, or the artificial
sweetener aspartame would be things to consider, she says. There's
another benefit, too. "The emotional burden of MS is huge, and if you
can get some sort of handle on it—there's something that you can
do?—that has a benefit as well. There's false hope and then there's
taking control," she says.

Here was the idea of control again.

WHY DO WE LIKE HAVING control so much? I ask Angela Duckworth,
a professor of psychology at the University of Pennsylvania who's

known for studying the importance of grit as a personality trait, which we'll explore later. She has a simple answer: "Usually when you don't have control bad things happen." This has been the case throughout human evolution. As a result, she says, "We are wired for control."

Experiment after experiment suggests that the absence of control leads to depression. Here's Angela Duckworth again: "When an animal experiences pain or adversity without being able to control it, the crucial thing is not the pain," she says of the research. "The crucial thing is the absence of control. Then subsequently they will demonstrate symptoms of depression. The idea is that if you have the expectancy that I can't do anything about this, then sort of the rational response is to not do anything." This idea, which we'll visit again later, became the basis for testing whether antidepressants worked or not: Researchers looked for whether a drug could prevent an animal from giving up if it thought it had no control over a negative situation.

Terry had never been one to think that she couldn't do anything about her situation. She took her doctor's advice and went to Ashton Embry's website.

A geology PhD who surveyed oil reserves in the Arctic for the Canadian government, Ashton Embry spent his free time rifling through published research that explored ideas outside the mainstream. He'd come to believe that traditional medicine was biased against answers that weren't pharmaceutical. He posted several studies on his site that suggested that a leaky gut was one of the culprits for MS.

Embry had become convinced that if you had leaky gut's sieve-like intestinal lining, the wrong things slipped into your system, triggering a sustained assault of inflammation. Like Char Walker, Embry believed eating the wrong foods led to this kind of permissive environment. And the wrong foods, according to Embry, were all the goodies you weren't allowed to eat on the Paleo diet.

The Paleo Diet

Proponents of the Paleo diet argue that humans just aren't built for grilled cheese. The Paleolithic era is generally thought to have started 2.6 million years ago (although there's some evidence that pushes the date back another 800,000 years). So over millions of years, our hunter-gatherer ancestors evolved on a diet of game, berries, nuts, tubers, and vegetables. Then, after the invention of agriculture, roughly 12,000 years ago, when we started feasting on grains, dairy, and beans, it was like putting unleaded gas in a diesel engine, the argument goes.

One critique of the diet is that our Paleolithic forebears lived only until fifty, on average, so we can't really make claims about their long-term health. "If Paleolithic people had lived longer, would they have gotten the common diseases we associate with old age? We just don't know," says Christina Warinner, a professor of anthropology and microbiome sciences at the University of Oklahoma and the Max Planck Institute for the Science of Human History. "We do know that [rates of] certain disorders, such as obesity and type 2 diabetes, have dramatically risen within the last few decades and this has nothing to do with the origins of agriculture," she says.

Loren Cordain, a professor emeritus of nutrition at Colorado State University, has written seven books on the Paleo diet, or The Paleo Diet™. (He trademarked the term.) Only a handful of small, short studies suggest that it may have a favorable impact on blood pressure, cholesterol, and body weight, among other factors. But while the evidence is so far very limited, Cordain says that specific components of the diet have been tested for more than a hundred years. "Say, for instance, the notion that refined carbohydrates and sugars have adverse health effects," he says. "Anybody that would say otherwise is a fool. It's one element of what Stone Age people did—they didn't eat refined sugars."

While we can be reasonably confident that there were no doughnuts in the Stone Age, other assumptions about the era are more problematic. Christina Warinner, the anthropologist, argues in her 2013

TEDx talk that the Paleo diet has no basis in the archaeological record. For one thing, scientists have discovered grains in the plaque on teeth of Paleolithic people and Neanderthals. She also points out that there was no single Paleolithic diet. Humans lived all over the world, and they ate what was locally available. So the Inuit people were eating a lot more sea mammals than their brethren to the landlocked south. Warinner also says that our fruits, vegetables, and animals—bred to be bigger, plumper, sweeter—barely resemble the sad, bitter, toxin-filled fare our forebears ate. The cabbage, kale, and brussels sprouts we eat today, for example, are more recent inventions.

Though history presents challenges to the Paleo philosophy, it is hard to argue with packing more fruits and vegetables into our diets. "If you remove wheat, cereal grains, and dairy from the diet, research shows that it actually increases the nutrient density of the diet," Loren Cordain tells me. "If you pull those food groups out, you get more vitamins, more minerals, more phytochemicals, and fiber." With fewer options, eaters are evidently forced into the available arms of produce—my family certainly was. That's an arrangement even the skeptical Christina Warinner can get behind. The lesson we can draw from the eating habits of Paleolithic people, Warinner says, is that we evolved to eat a great variety of whole foods and to eat them when they're fresh and in season. No preservatives, no additives, no processed foods.

People in developing countries still eat this way—and they don't get autoimmune diseases like we do in the industrialized world, says Mass General's Dr. Fasano. The hygiene hypothesis emerged to explain this difference. Because our high rates of autoimmune diseases coincided with better hygiene and a drop in infections, perhaps our immune systems, primed for millennia to fight off constant attacks, were overreacting now that they were exposed to fewer enemies. People in developing countries, where hygiene was suboptimal, had high rates of infection but seemed to be protected from the onslaught of autoimmune disease.

That's the theory. But in countries where the hygiene has improved, in North Africa and some South American countries, we don't see infections like we used to, says Dr. Fasano. We don't see autoimmune diseases, either. But if these people migrate to industrialized countries, they get the same kind of risk that we do. "So something else is going on, and I believe diet is the key element," Dr. Fasano says. "We don't eat the way we used to."

We've changed the way we eat faster than our bodies have evolved to handle it, says Dr. Fasano. He points out that humans ate a certain way for millions of years, and in this last century alone our diets have changed radically. "Think of this: 2.6 million years that we lived that way," he says of our hunter-gatherer tradition. "The refrigerator was invented only three generations ago. Only three generations ago!" he says.

This was ultimately Terry Wahls's takeaway about diet: She needed to concentrate on whole fruits and vegetables because the typical Western diet doesn't supply nearly enough nutrients.

When she first adopted the Paleo diet years before, she'd been focused on what she needed to take out: the grains, dairy, sugar, and legumes that she believed could lead to a leaky gut. This had been one of the themes of Ashton Embry's website, and it still made sense to her. Now, she realized, she also needed to add in more beneficial food. It was a two-pronged strategy—continue to try to avoid a leaky gut and also deluge her mitochondria with the nutrients they needed.

She started eating twelve cups a day of berries and vegetables, packing in all the heavies—beets, mushrooms, broccoli, blueberries, cabbage, and, of course, kale, that nutritional ingenue. She made sure she got a variety of greens and deeply colored produce. She sprinkled nutrient-dense kelp powder and green tea extract on her meals. The richness of her new diet allowed her to cut back on some of her supplements. She also embraced nuts, avocados, coconut milk, and coconut oil for their fats. As an established adherent to the Paleo diet, she already knew how rewarding a relationship with bacon could be. Grass-fed beef and oily fish, too, which supplied valuable omega-3s. Organ meat was especially efficient, a full house, crowded with vitamins.

"That's when the magic happened," she says.

✿   ✿   ✿

OVER THE NEXT YEAR, TERRY'S strength came home to her. She ditched her reclining wheelchair for an upright electric scooter. Then she even started parking that at the door of the clinic and using a cane to walk between exam rooms—her feet made friends with the ground again. It had been five years since she'd set out to slow her disease down.

Eating well isn't convenient. Cramming in that many fresh vegetables takes a lot of effort, and Terry's whole family pitched in to make it work.

Here's how the day went. Terry would be up at five-thirty for a tall glass of blenderized greens and a half hour of isometric exercises hooked up to her e-stim machine. Before leaving for work she'd dump a heap of chopped vegetables and meat in the Crock-Pot for dinner— sweet potatoes, onions, cabbage, and ground bison, perhaps, sprinkled with kelp powder, spices, and sea salt. Jackie took care of the shopping. When Terry got home from work, by six, she'd take up her station on a stool in the kitchen, orchestrating the rest of the dinner, usually a massive pile of greens. Zach and Zebby did most of the washing and chopping. After dinner, Terry crammed in a half hour each of more isometrics and strength training with weights while the kids and Jackie cleaned up. Then Terry would lay out the vegetables that needed to be prepped for the next night's slow-cooked stew, and the kids would engage their knives again.

One day, four months into her twelve-cup-a-day diet, Terry was scheduled to meet with her boss, Dr. Paul Rothman, for her annual review. It was early spring 2008. His office was up a big hill so she headed out for the appointment on her scooter. Halfway up the slope, the battery died on her. Fuming at herself for not having left earlier, she got off the scooter and started pushing it up the hill. At the top, she found a campus shuttle stop, but the next bus wasn't going to come for another half hour. She checked her watch. She was already twenty minutes late. She didn't have time to wait for the shuttle, so she abandoned her scooter and pressed on.

When she finally got to Dr. Rothman's office, his secretary scolded her. Terry remembers her saying, "Where have you been?" Terry was flustered and apologetic as she walked in to face the chief of medicine. When he saw her, he didn't say anything. He wasn't annoyed; he had no words.

The last time he'd seen her, about a year before, she'd been lifeless in her wheelchair, barely able to hold her head up. She had little use of her arms. She looked so ill, he tells me, he was concerned about her ability to survive. "And then to see her walk in . . ." Dr. Rothman says. "I mean, it was holy cow. I'll never forget it."

For her part, Terry was so concerned about being late that she hadn't noticed that she'd just accomplished a major physical task.

They'd been scheduled to discuss her job performance, but they didn't get to it that day. Dr. Rothman told Terry that she needed to have a case report written up immediately on herself, the usual first step for procuring research funding. She needed to find out whether what she'd done would work on anyone else.

At home, her transformation was more difficult to grasp. While everyone in the family was certainly aware of her increased mobility, they had little faith that it was more than a last hurrah on a downward trip, a quirk of a reliably confounding disease. She still had a degenerative illness, one you didn't come back from as far as anyone knew.

Zach never stopped thinking that his mother would have to quit working in two years. He just didn't buy that she was actually recovering, and certainly not by eating particular foods. "You just have to change your diet?" he says now with a pretend scoff. He'd won a scholarship to study in Germany for a year after high school, which he'd forfeited during his mom's upswing, in part for fear that something would happen to her health while he was away. He told his mom it was because he didn't want to be away from his girlfriend.

You may have seen Zach Wahls before. In 2011, he stood up to speak at a public forum on gay marriage at the Iowa House of Representatives. The then-nineteen-year-old told the lawmakers that his family wasn't so different from any other Iowa family. The clip of his three-minute speech has been viewed over eighteen million times on YouTube. The online phenomenon led to a book deal, a speech at the Democratic National Convention, and an introduction to President Obama. The book, *My Two Moms: Lessons of Love, Strength, and What Makes a Family,* was published in 2012.

ONE SATURDAY MORNING IN 2008, Zach was in the kitchen when he heard Zebby yelling in the garage. He opened the door. Terry was reaching for a bike helmet. Zebby was saying, "You're out of your goddamned mind."

Zach was more measured. "Mom," he said, "you've got to be careful. It's a little different now."

She and Jackie used to enjoy twenty-mile rides together. But as her MS progressed it had stolen her balance. By the time Zebby was making a fuss in the garage, it had been six years since Terry had been on a bike.

Here's what happened: Terry, confident as usual, is saying, "I think I'm okay. I think today's the day." And by now Jackie has come out, and she starts lowering the seat on Terry's old Trek bike, which Zach had been using.

They all walk down the driveway to the street. Zach helps his mother get her leg over the bar since her balance was still a little iffy. Both he and Zebby take up positions on either side of her. As her feet press on the pedals, the kids start running to keep up with their mother. Zach is ready to push her toward the grass for a softer fall if he sees her wobble.

And then she goes.

Her children and Jackie cheered like parents who'd just taken the training wheels off and let go of their six-year-old's bike for the first time. But it was the reverse, of course, of that rite of passage, the children moved to see their mom make it on her own. They were all crying. "That moment means more to me than almost anything else I've ever experienced," says Zach. "Seeing my mom on the bike." There are layers of wonder. Wonder at the fact that she could ride a bike again. And wonder that such a regular act could be wondrous.

All those months that Terry had been feeling better, she never believed that real recovery was possible, either. But after that day on the bike she thought: *Well, no one really knows.*

5

Diet and Inflammation

Terry Looks for Proof

AFTER SHE FIRST RECOVERED, TERRY GOT TO WORK ON HER CASE study, in addition to continuing to teach primary care residents and seeing patients in the brain trauma clinic at the VA hospital.

Next she wrote grant proposals to try to get her entire protocol tested—the mounds of vegetables, the meats, the berries, the powdered thises and thats, the kit, the caboodle, and the neuromuscular electrical stimulation. The whole messy thing at once.

But scientists don't do messy, particularly those who fund studies. They want to know what single molecule you're testing, and they want to know the mechanism—exactly how it works. After all, how can you tell which factor, or combination of factors, have an effect if you test them all at once? Terry wanted to bake the entire cake to see if it would turn out well again, whereas science usually cued in on a single ingredient at a time. And she couldn't explain exactly how she'd gotten better. The only thing she knew for sure was that she had.

Competition for NIH funding is extremely stiff. The joke among biomedical researchers is that you already need to have proven your results before you can get a grant. "They don't want to fund you if they're not sure you'll be successful," says Veena Taneja, the researcher and associate professor of immunology at the Mayo Clinic. "It's absurd because you have to do something before you know whether this will work or not."

The NIH turned down Terry's grant application, as did the MS Society, which funds tens of millions of dollars of research a year. She knew what the science rules were. She'd just come to believe they were dumb. The traditional approach, she thought, was overly concerned with isolating a single factor and identifying the mechanism. That model was fine if you were testing a pharmaceutical, but diet, which is a kaleidoscope of molecules, required a less militaristic approach. And since cutting out bagels wasn't exactly high risk, she thought looser study standards should be acceptable.

When Terry's proposal was rejected, it was like being dumped by someone she didn't even like. That said, she would have been happy marrying either institution for the money to fund her research.

It was clear that if she was going to get financial support for her work, it was not going to come from the usual sources. In 2009, she flew up to Calgary to meet with Ashton Embry, the geologist whose son had MS. In addition to maintaining his website, he had started a foundation, Direct-MS, to fund outside-the-box research.

The Direct-MS board agreed to help fund the cost of her trial, writing her a check for $56,000. At the same time, the manufacturer of Terry's e-stim machine donated $40,000 worth of devices. The University of Iowa kicked in labor: A couple of undergraduates got credit for working on the study.

By the time she enrolled thirteen people with progressive MS to test her protocol, it went beyond the vegetable-heavy diet plus supplements and electrical stimulation. The list also included strengthening exercises, stretches, massage, and meditation. Participants would remain on their medications.

The protocol was a lot to keep up with, especially when fatigue was an issue. Right away, three participants failed to stick to the diet for seven days and so were dropped. Ten remained.

Eight people ended up completing twelve months on the protocol, and they showed "significant improvement in fatigue," she and her research team wrote in one paper.

Once she demonstrated that the protocol was safe, she was cleared to bump up the number of participants in the trial to twenty. The Direct-MS board wrote another check to cover the cost of MRI (magnetic resonance imaging) for the additional people. More support came through her newly created Wahls Foundation, which paid the salary of a PhD student who worked on the trial, and covered the cost of extending it for two more years.

Of the nineteen people who made it through twelve months on the protocol, eleven were considered "high responders," according to a second paper. They showed a "clinically significant decrease" in their perceived fatigue. It's important to remember that the trial did not include a control group, so it's impossible to rule out the placebo effect. Fatigue is also difficult to measure objectively.

Terry's team also looked at how well their study participants could walk, taking videos of them before they started the protocol and at regular intervals throughout the trial. Because Terry's paper summing up the data is still under review, it is too soon to report those results. But she couldn't resist showing me a number of the videos and gave me permission to share what I saw: Some of the participants showed a dramatic improvement in walking ability and speed. Their mood, cognition, brain structure, and quality of life were also measured, and that data is being analyzed now.

Annette Reed was the first patient Terry enrolled. When I spoke to Reed, she was forty-eight; she had been diagnosed with MS eight years before. She had never gotten the sense that her neurologists could do much to help her. One of them once held out three medications in his hands and told her to pick one. *Really?* she thought but didn't say. Having MS, she told me, "is a scary thing and you don't know what your options are and slowly you go downhill."

By the time she went to hear Terry speak about MS at the local Unitarian church, Reed had lost a lot of function on her left side and was struggling to walk. She would get wiped out after doing the dishes for five minutes and need to take a break. And she was just beginning to feel her right side start to go. *If I lose my right side, I'm S.O.L.*, thought Reed, who's married and owns her own travel agency. At her last visit to the neurologist, he said he was going to start her on a chemo drug, which terrified her.

That day at the church, Terry told her about her upcoming diet-and-everything-else trial. "I'll never forget this," Reed told me. "We were all sitting at these tables. She squatted in front of me for fifteen minutes." Reed thought, *Okay, if you can do that on the protocol, let's talk.*

On Terry's protocol, Reed's fatigue left town. It was still absent three years later when we spoke. That wasn't all. The pain, the stiffness, and the spasms, all of those symptoms were gone. Fixing the walking, though, has been tougher. She is improving but very slowly. That her downward trajectory has been tilted upward at all is remarkable. She uses a walk aid, a cuff below her knee that stimulates a muscle contraction to help her raise her foot. "The hope is that one day I'll be able to get rid of it," she said. That's not the kind of optimism progressive MS patients are generally taught to have.

But however positive Terry's outcomes are, diet studies like hers are still considered somewhat unreliable. Because until scientists figure out a way to put kale in disguise, it's going to be very hard to design a double-blind, placebo-controlled study. Fake electrical stimulation seems tricky, too, but may be doable. Plus, Terry didn't have enough funding to study more people—and statistically it's difficult to show anything with just ten or even twenty people, especially without a control group.

Another strike against Terry's trial is that the data couldn't be collected entirely in the lab because asking volunteers to be locked up for years and fed all their meals is a bit of a hard sell. So Terry, like most people who study diet, has had to rely on self-reporting—people in the study kept journals of what they ate. The problem is that getting people to document everything they put into their bodies can be more confessional than scientific. Terry is the first to admit that relying on patients to do the reporting is not an ideal way to obtain information. In fact, one study subject went on a pizza bender and failed to include that detail in her notebook. She ended up coming clean about it later in conversation with Terry. But you go to war with the study you have.

So there are legitimate reasons why nutrition studies tend to be the unloved stepsisters of pharmaceutical trials. From this perspective, the MS Society's dismissal of Terry's proposal was understandable. But in the handful of years since the group rejected her grant proposal, the organization has undergone a shift.

The MS Society has been tracking the evolving science of diet and inflammation. At the same time the group has kept a close watch on social media and surveyed its own constituents about what matters to them. It's clear that interest in lifestyle interventions, including diet and exercise, is high. "Because it's of such importance to people with MS, we have made it a priority," says Kathleen Costello, the organization's vice president for healthcare access. "There is some evidence to believe that diet may have an important role in MS. There's keen interest from the research community to explore the inflammatory process in relation to food," she says. But just as crucial: "We try very hard to listen to what our constituents say." And they want answers.

Which is how in 2014, Terry got a call inviting her to participate in the National MS Society's first-ever wellness meeting, to talk about the effect of diet and exercise and other non-pharmaceutical interventions. Terry was so stunned that she asked if they were sure. The real kicker, she says, was at the meeting itself, when one of the research officers asked her to resubmit her grant proposal, promising to go back and forth with her to make it fit their criteria.

Still, Terry's story remains controversial. In 2011, she gave a talk at TEDx Iowa City—a kind of grassroots TED that falls outside the curatorial jurisdiction of the official organization. The clip is posted on

YouTube, but there's a warning from big TED distancing itself from the material since it's advice based on a personal narrative. As with a racy movie, viewer discretion is advised.

The nutrition expert, Loren Cordain, makes clear that he isn't a fan of Terry's—even though he's a proponent of the Paleo diet. "I don't think she's a scientist by any means. I don't think she really understands how and why what she's doing may be therapeutic for MS patients," he says. Terry responds that he's absolutely right, which is why she's so keen on more study.

WITH SUCH UNUSUAL SUCCESS, AN obvious question is whether Terry actually had MS to begin with. Her current neurologist, Dr. Ezzatollah Shivapour, tells me that while there are no absolutes, MRI and spinal fluid analysis, both of which Terry has had, allow him to be over 95 percent certain that she has MS. Also, blood tests have ruled out other diseases that mimic MS, says Dr. Shivapour, who spoke to me with Terry's permission.

Perhaps, I ask, she hadn't actually transitioned to the secondary-progressive classification and her recovery is part of the cycle you expect to see with relapsing-remitting patients? Dr. Shivapour, who specializes in MS and is a clinical professor of neurology at the University of Iowa Carver College of Medicine, tells me that while there are no tests for it, Terry's clinical presentation, going back to 2005, was most consistent with secondary-progressive MS; she had been declining steadily and steeply. He is as sure about the secondary-progressive part as he is about the MS diagnosis, which is as sure as any neurologist can be, he says.

He has been happy to watch Terry improve, but he also wants to be clear that her recovery is not a recovery from paralysis: She never lost the use of her legs. It irritates him to hear her described as having cured herself of MS. "That is just nonsense. We don't have a cure for anything," he says.

When Terry was working on her book about her interventions—
The Wahls Protocol, published in 2014—she would send Dr. Shivapour

copies of the manuscript for review. His note was: "Try to not exaggerate to the extent that people think that, 'My God! She was paralyzed and incontinent and a vegetable and now she's walking!' Because this is not going to happen." For the record, he does not think that she exaggerates. But she does talk about her protocol with such absolute sureness—with none of the scientist's skepticism given that the data is thin—that you can see how he could be wary.

No doubt about it, though, she has recovered, he says. That's the word he uses. "The person who goes from a scooter to a stick to me is recovery. The person who goes from a walker to a stick is recovery. She has recovered reasonably well and remains physically independent from any assistive device," he says.

When I meet Terry, her gait appears completely normal, though she tells me that it does tend to deteriorate somewhat as the day wears on. And she still gets tired, she says. Maybe, but that same evening, when I'm ready to collapse at my hotel after spending the day with her, Terry insists on demonstrating her workout routine. Once she built her muscles back up with electrical stimulation, she substituted exercise to maintain her strength. She no longer needs the e-stim machine. These days she spends a full hour a day doing some combination of swimming, biking, strength training, yoga, Pilates, tae kwon do kicks, and stretching.

In consultation with Dr. Shivapour, Terry tapered off most of her medications in 2008, once she was lifting weights, walking around, and biking again. She has stayed on one—gabapentin—for the zinging facial pain. "I don't have the nerve to go off it," she says. And the pain still comes, though just a couple of times a year now. She can quiet those flare-ups quickly and effectively with oral prednisone, a steroid.

She makes a point of telling me that she hasn't cured her MS. But she is better. Clearly.

Although empirically we can't know for sure why, Dr. Shivapour credits her protocol. In fact, he's a coauthor of two published papers drawn from Terry's original trial. The people who did well, he says, are the ones who were the most committed to the diet, electrical stimulation, and exercise plan. Those whose symptoms progressed are the ones who did not keep up with the program, Dr. Shivapour says.

He is sympathetic. "It's a really restrictive diet," he says. "I couldn't do it myself. You need to have nine servings of fruits and vegetables a day." (Terry lowered the intake from twelve to nine cups to make it more doable for other people.) Dr. Shivapour goes on: "I hate kale. My wife tries to make it in different ways. Every time we go to the farmers' market, my wife buys kale. She sneaks bits of it into meals. I'm like a child. I say, 'Did you put kale in here?'" And it's a lot harder to stick with anything when you're tired or depressed or don't have family support. "So," he says, "they don't really do the exercises or use the machine as they're supposed to." Wasn't it more than enough just to have MS?

Dr. Shivapour says it's not a stretch to believe the plan could work because it's based on factors that are already known to be good for us. "Everyone knows physical exercise is good," he says. "If I put you in bed for three months and get you out and say 'Go ahead and run,' you cannot because you're deconditioned. So the body needs to be physically active. Everyone knows a good diet is good for you even if you have diabetes or cancer or depression. Everyone knows that neuromuscular electrical stimulation helps [restore strength]. They use that with broken bones, for deconditioned patients, muscle weakness, and atrophy. So everyone knows those three elements work." But until Terry, as far as anyone knows, no one had ever taken each component so far and put them all together.

It still seems a little outrageous to suggest that you could tackle a disease like MS by eating vegetables, taking supplements, exercising, getting electrical stimulation, stretching, meditating, *getting a massage.* How could the answer not be more of a heavyweight?

I call Dr. M. Flint Beal, professor of neurology and neuroscience at Weill Cornell Medical College in New York City, who'd written the paper about the mice and the mitochondria that had been so inspiring to Terry. I tell him, I know a woman who has MS and was using a wheelchair because her fatigue had become so debilitating, and she read your paper about how our cells' mitochondria are a factor in Parkinson's disease and that by supporting the mitochondria with certain nutrients the mice in your study got better, so she started taking what your mice took and, well, now she doesn't need to use a wheelchair anymore. I ask him, Does that make any sense at all to you?

"Uh," he says. "Yes." He explains: "The thing we were trying to potentially modify was mitochondrial impairment and oxidative damage and I think those are part of the pathogenesis of MS. There is a substantial body of literature that suggests that MS can be associated with mitochondrial defects."

What about the big list of vitamins Terry came up with to benefit her mitochondria? He can see how that could work? "Yes," he says again. "There are a lot of things that have been shown to have some beneficial effects, but mostly in vitro or in small-animal studies. I think it's feasible that it could work in MS."

THE THING I WONDER ABOUT Terry is, what made her think she'd be able to figure out a plan, on her own, from her recliner at night while her kids were in bed, when the top researchers were stumped? It was pretty nervy.

When you spend time with Terry, you get to know her ego well. It's as tall as she is. But she got herself out of a wheelchair. She *is* hot shit. I ask her what the future looks like to her. She's not too shy to suggest the Nobel.

One night, after I have dinner with her family, Terry takes me on a tour of the basement of their Iowa City home. Pictures of Jackie and the children and Zach's trophies look out from shelves, but the walls are all Terry. Here is an album cover–size photograph of her in full tae kwon do regalia doing a high kick off the side of a mountain. Here she is in a cross-country ski race. Here is a self-portrait she did in college. And another one. And another. Taking me by one more, she says, this basement docent, "So, a lot of promise. Also a lot to do."

Many of us, myself included, might naturally recoil from such outsize self-worth. But meeting Terry changed how I think about big egos. Not only do I feel she's earned hers, but I wonder if she could have been extraordinarily bold without it.

If she were more entrenched in the mainstream, in regular thinking, she probably would have figured that as a clinician who had never done any research, she wasn't likely to come up with a way to recover from her own incurable disease. Certainly she wasn't just going to puzzle it out in her head. And yet that's what she did. A more reasonable person would have been persuaded by the odds. A more reasonable person would have assumed her doctors knew more about MS than she did. A more reasonable person would still be using a wheelchair.

POSTSCRIPT: IN AUGUST 2016, THE National MS Society committed over $1 million to study the effect of Terry's diet on MS-related fatigue compared to a low-saturated-fat diet.

6

The Science of Success

What Makes Us Try and Try Again

WHAT MADE TERRY WAHLS DIFFERENT FROM MOST PEOPLE? What made her, along with others in this book, think their own actions could change what was likely to be unchangeable?

I asked this question of Angela Duckworth, the University of Pennsylvania professor of psychology who coined the term "grit," which she defines as perseverance and passion for very long-term goals. On the heels of a popular TED talk about the concept, she wrote *Grit: The Power of Passion and Perseverance.* She says that grit stands out as a major predictor of success—more than IQ, more than social intelligence, more than family background. Among West Point cadets, national spelling bee contestants, salespeople, teachers, and students, according to Duckworth's research, the ones who do well share this one quality: They're persistent. And being persistent works.

Terry and others in these pages, with their exceptional, almost crazy determination, bear this out.

But how did they get that way? What makes a person gritty, be indomitable? We don't know yet, says Duckworth. It's one of the questions she's hoping to tackle through more research at Penn's Character Lab, where she's the founder and scientific director.

Although science is still figuring out why people become resolute, Duckworth says one way to try to understand motivation is to look at the rational agent model of economics. The idea is that people will try to do things that seem likely to work out and are good for them and not bad for them. The thing is, we all calculate these values differently. People have individual interpretations of what constitutes a long shot or a jackpot.

Duckworth uses an entrepreneur to illustrate the variability that impacts motivation. Say someone worked for fifteen years on developing a transistor, a device used in electronics. From the outside, you might look at that effort at the start, calculate the probability of success and the potential payoff, and come to the conclusion that the entrepreneur is out of his mind. But Duckworth thinks that from the perspective of the entrepreneur, the extended effort is completely rational. The stereotype is that entrepreneurs are risk-loving. "It's actually not the case," she says. They just see better odds of success. Particularly if they are self-confident.

The value of the payoff can be just as subjective. "When you look at really gritty people, like Nobel laureates, the payoffs for them are in the currency of interest and purpose," says Duckworth. In other words, the payoff is a sense of meaning. And the value of meaning, of that form of compensation, is much higher than people on the outside can appreciate.

Though she hasn't directly studied persistence in the face of a health problem, she says, "For a parent, I think, to have something that is meaningful or relevant or consequential for our children might trump everything. It's wired"—it's in our makeup as humans. "The payoff," Duckworth says, "is infinite." This is certainly how I experienced it.

Another key factor of what Duckworth calls grit, of course, is hard work. This, too, is another variable. People have very different subjective experiences of effort, she says. "We find, for example, that really gritty people don't experience really hard practice as aversively as other people do. For many of them the costs are actually lower. Really gritty people eventually learn to do highly effortful things without the subjective cost."

But none of this works if there isn't also hope. There's no grit without it.

That's because, as Duckworth is quoted as saying in Terry Wahls's chapter, if you expect that you can't do anything about your situation, then the rational response is not to do anything. "You have to maintain hope," she says. "So what is hope? Basically, the idea of hope is the expectancy that there's something I can do to improve my situation and one of the things that would make you lose hope is to perceive that you can't."

And your perception is informed by your life history, Duckworth says. Referring to the people in this book, she says, "What in their life have they learned? [What taught them] that if you keep working at something, it will work out? That basic insight—if you want to take hope one level deeper, if you want to lift up the hood on hope—is about expectations that you can do something. And that in part is influenced by your history of being exposed to situations where you can do something or not."

This seems like a possible explanation for why the people in this book are so resilient. Everyone here has a history of agency, of *doing something*—and of succeeding as a result. Many of them had difficult childhoods or faced other adversity that they overcame before having to confront illness.

Certainly genes can't be discounted—and Terry seemed determined from the get-go.

So did Amanda Hanson, a mother you're about to meet.

7

Amanda Hanson

Love and Sacrifice

My God, we went through all of that. We can't fall apart now.
—Bryan and Amanda Hanson

Hayden was a baby when his body started choking itself.
He had just tried solid food for the first time: barley cereal, which the
pediatrician had recommended over the usual rice variety for its
added nutritional punch. A first-time mom, Amanda Hanson had
made a production of feeding Hayden spoonfuls; each one was a plane
buzzing on approach to the landing field of his mouth, turning it into
a big, gummy smile. He was an easy baby. He had dark brown eyes
and a little bit of fuzzy hair that matched them. He was always stretching his arms out on either side of him in an expression that seemed to
say, "I'm so happy!"

After lunch, the two set out in the car to do some errands in Brain-
tree, their quiet suburb close to Boston. As she was driving, Amanda
heard a strange coughing sound behind her. She turned around; her

son's face was hidden by his rear-facing seat. By the time Amanda pulled in to a Target parking lot, Hayden was struggling to breathe. She grabbed his body and started running. She crashed through the doors of the store, yelling for someone to call 911.

The ambulance came quickly. Hayden lay on a bench as a paramedic scissored open his gray fleece hoodie from wrist to shoulder. Hayden's eyes were swollen shut and hives bloomed across the folds of his soft skin. The bridge of his nose widened as if he'd had botched plastic surgery. He was going into anaphylaxis, a severe allergic reaction to the barley, which can interfere with the ability to breathe.

Amanda already understood that her baby's immune system had made a disastrously wrong call and was overreacting: It had registered barley as dangerous and had mounted an allergic assault that was so aggressive that it threatened his life. If the response wasn't checked, he could end up being killed by his own act of self-protection—like a honeybee, dying because it used its stinger.

An IV of epinephrine, which works in part by relaxing the muscles in the airways, was slipped into the pudge of his arm. Hayden was loaded into the ambulance, his little body strapped down to an adult-size gurney. A tiny breathing mask muffled his crying. His blood pressure finally stabilized, but his features seemed to keep melting into his face. Amanda, frantic, tried to reach her husband, Bryan, but he was in China on a business trip and didn't pick up. This would come to seem like a refrain in her life—Hayden in danger, and she was on her own to try to help him.

Amanda looked down at her son. If he reacted this way to something as innocuous as baby cereal, she wondered in horror what the extent of his allergies might be.

Amanda herself had grown up with allergies, to tree nuts. In fact, she had her own EpiPen with her that day—an emergency dose of epinephrine—but she didn't think it would be safe to use it on Hayden.

At Boston Children's Hospital, Amanda began to get a sense of what her family was in for. Blood tests indicated that Hayden was highly sensitive to a number of different foods. The results meant that he had an elevated risk of having an allergic reaction to them. At that point only the barley allergy was definitive because he had experienced symptoms in addition to testing positive. Even so, Hayden would have to avoid eating wheat, milk, eggs, peanuts, tree nuts, and rye, too.

"It was overwhelming," says Amanda. "I remember feeling like they were putting a pillow over my face." And Hayden had been tested for only the most common allergies. Over the next couple of years the number of foods Hayden needed to avoid would eventually stretch to twenty-eight.

Amanda had always planned to go back to work while Hayden was still young. Before becoming pregnant, she'd completed her PhD in psychology and begun the hundreds of postdoctoral training hours she needed to finish before becoming a therapist. Once Hayden was diagnosed with such severe allergies, though, Amanda wasn't comfortable leaving him with anyone else. She let go of her own plans. Hayden's allergies became her job instead.

In this new occupation she was no less ambitious than she had been in psychology. Amanda had personal drive to spare, and she put it all into protecting Hayden. She would be the toughest, the strongest, the best. Because Hayden's allergies weren't really a job, after all. They were a calling.

IF YOU'RE DIAGNOSED WITH FOOD allergies today, the only thing your doctor can do for you is tell you the diagnosis. The prescription is to stay away from the offending food and to keep an EpiPen with you at all times in case you're accidentally exposed. There is always the hope that a child will outgrow his or her food allergies, but despite some promising research, there is no cure and no preventive medication.

Avoiding certain foods is a straightforward enough command that's very hard to follow. Just six months after his first ambulance ride, Hayden's throat was squeezing off his breath again. The family had recently moved into a new house. A couple with a baby girl came over to welcome them to the neighborhood. While Amanda and Bryan chatted with the parents at the door, the one-year-old girl spotted Hayden inside by the toy bin and tottered over.

It happened fast. Amanda heard a sound. When she found Hayden, he was projectile vomiting and couldn't stop. He'd grabbed the girl's sippy cup and taken a drink. Amanda saw that there was a drop of chocolate milk on the corner of his mouth.

By the time Hayden was nine, he would struggle against death six more times. For Amanda and Bryan, anaphylaxis was a horror movie, an invisible hand closing around their son's throat. Like all parents of allergic children, they were always armed with an EpiPen so that they could administer its lifesaving shot of epinephrine themselves if they had to. The key was to do it right away, to stop the reaction before Hayden suffocated. Amanda once pulled Hayden's pants down in the middle of a Friendly's parking lot to give him a shot in the thigh.

Despite the urgency, it was still difficult *not* to hesitate because using an EpiPen required using considerable force to stab a needle into an already terrified child. There was even a period when Hayden would run away from his parents in that moment. As necessary as the EpiPen was, it felt like trauma heaped on trauma. You wanted to use it only if you had to, and, given the stakes, it was always preferable to get to a hospital. Using an EpiPen is also no guarantee that the allergic reaction will be stopped. In 2013, a thirteen-year-old girl died from an allergic reaction after eating a snack that contained peanuts, even though three EpiPens were administered.

For Amanda, the stress of the rescues was cumulative, and there was no relief from the constant sense of peril. Taking care of Hayden during the day, Amanda had to be on heightened alert, a threat advisory scale always set to red.

And then there was the constant problem of coming up with good meals for Hayden. He would end up eating chicken with rice four nights a week. He was always in the bottom 5th percentile for height and weight for his age group. Some days Amanda would be trolling the grocery store looking for food her son could eat, reading lists of ingredients, and she would break down in the middle of the aisle, crying. Once she abandoned her shopping cart and just went home.

They had recently moved from California, and Amanda had no friends. "I remember just feeling so isolated," she says.

She regularly checked the websites of various allergy organizations for news and guidance. One of them sponsored a support group for parents of children with food allergies, and Amanda started going. "Don't you get so frustrated when you see the kids on the monkey bars and they've just eaten a peanut butter sandwich?" someone would say, inducing nodding all around, a room full of bobble-head moms. More than anything, they shared cooking advice. "Okay, my kid is allergic to wheat, dairy, and eggs," another mom would say. "Anybody have a muffin recipe?"

At one of those meetings, the word went around that the chef Ming Tsai was looking for adults with food allergies to appear on his TV cooking show. Tsai's young son had food allergies, and the chef wanted to raise awareness about the problem. Amanda volunteered— her allergy to tree nuts. So one night she and Bryan went to Blue Ginger, Tsai's Wellesley, Massachusetts, restaurant, to tape a segment about how to order safely.

After they ordered a fake dinner for the cameras, Amanda and Bryan were having a glass of wine when Tsai came over to thank them. Amanda mentioned her own son's allergies. "Hey," Tsai said, "for what it's worth, my wife is taking our son to this healer. He just started the treatment but we're having some pretty positive results already."

By that point—Hayden was four—they'd heard about a lot of supposed wonder cures and had attempted most of them. Acupressure, chiropractic, something called NAET, which stands for Nambudripad's Allergy Elimination Techniques. Nothing had ever worked on Hayden or on anyone they knew. Bryan figured that if Tsai's son was having any luck, his allergies couldn't have been as severe as Hayden's; whatever it was this so-called healer was doing would never work for his own son. As for Amanda, her own hope had taken on the pallor of desperation. *You want me to stand on my head twenty-three of the twenty-four hours a day?* she thought. *I'll do it. I'll grasp on to anything.*

Amanda made an appointment. The healer was a woman named Amy Thieringer, who saw clients out of a physical therapist's office. A single mother with three small children, Thieringer had just opened her own practice for treating allergies. She used a very unconventional approach, which she'd developed herself.

Thieringer said that Hayden was having allergic reactions because his immune system was "overloaded" from things such as infections or environmental toxins. In this "heightened state" it was overreacting, even to something as innocent as food. Thieringer tried to explain that this was creating blockages in his energy pathways. To help Hayden get better, to get his body not to have allergic reactions, she needed to "balance his immune system," Thieringer said.

To see what was overloading his system—step 1 of a complex therapy program—Thieringer had Hayden take hold of a metal wand that was connected by a cord to a small device. This was Thieringer's Bio-Scan machine, which was about the size of a box that could hold a pair of children's boots and sat on her desktop. It was linked to a laptop. As Hayden held the wand in his right hand—it looked more like a brass jump rope handle—Thieringer took hold of an implement herself, which she called a stylus. It resembled a fat writing pen, had a brass tip, and was also connected to the BioScan machine. Thieringer then pressed the tip of the stylus to a spot on Hayden's left pointer finger. This site on his finger, she said, was a portal into his network of energy pathways.

A weak electrical current was then released through the stylus into Hayden's finger. Thieringer said that the machine measured how quickly the electricity made the trip through the closed circuit from the stylus past the portal in Hayden's finger, through his energy corridors, and back out again to the wand. By looking at the flow of energy between the two points, she said she could see whether his system was balanced or not, and which environmental allergens, such as mold or dust, Hayden was sensitive to.

To restore balance, Thieringer used several different approaches, some of which tapped into the mind and were based on various anxiety therapies. Once Hayden's immune system was balanced, Thieringer could begin to reintroduce foods safely, she said, in gradually increasing amounts, everything Hayden had been allergic to.

Energy pathways? A portal? A *wand? How in God's name,* Amanda thought, *is this thing hooked up to a computer going to possibly change his internal system? This is a bunch of hokeypokey. This is . . . wow.*

But she went back. "I was totally desperate. That's what it takes. You almost have to be on the brink of losing it to be a pioneer in this," she tells me.

They saw Thieringer for two more sessions before Bryan got a promotion and the family left Massachusetts for Boulder, Colorado. There'd been no change in Hayden, and Amanda wasn't broken up about quitting. "I thought, 'Eh, it probably wouldn't have worked anyway.'"

When Hayden turned five and started kindergarten, it became harder to protect him. He started to be invited to birthday parties, and he had his own ideas about which kids he wanted to have playdates with. In Massachusetts, Amanda had always arranged them with moms from the support group.

But before Amanda and Bryan could let Hayden venture out into his life, they had to teach him about death. They told him that it could happen if he wasn't careful about every bite he took. While he was five, six, and seven, Amanda and Bryan told me, they were using the word "die" regularly. Before field trips, Amanda said to him, "Honey, if somebody has a bag of candy on the bus and they turn around and offer you a piece, you can't have it even if it's a candy you know you can have. You can't because it could have touched something else, and you could die." Hayden would respond, "Okay, Mom. Okay."

Bryan tells me, "At that young age, he had a realization that he could die. And I think not many kids ever think about it. But he understood." While Hayden was in school, Amanda always stayed within a two-mile radius. "I was scared I'd get that phone call: 'Something happened at lunch. . . .'" By second grade, he had his own cellphone.

*   *   *

AMANDA AND BRYAN MET ON an airplane. It was 1994. They'd first noticed each other in the Toledo, Ohio, terminal, waiting for a flight to Chicago. He was in town for a business meeting. She was a senior at Bowling Green State, going to visit grad schools for psychology. "I remember I had a newspaper with me," Bryan tells me. "She was across the way. We kind of looked at each other, held eyes for a little bit." But she was with a guy, so he went back to reading the paper. Once on board, Bryan was taking off his coat, getting situated, when he noticed that she'd gotten on alone. There were three open seats, one of which was next to her.

After the plane took off, Bryan walked up and asked if the seat was taken. "I sat down and didn't say anything else," says Bryan. Amanda was too busy thinking, *Oh my gosh he's so cute,* to open her mouth. (The guy in the terminal was a friend.) "It was a very short flight so I knew if I was going to say something I had to say something," says Bryan. He was working on some sales figures on his laptop. And so, like so many Casanovas before him, he asked her which spreadsheet looked better. "Clearly he was not a player. I was able to spot those guys with the rehearsed one-liners," Amanda says. "He was so nervous. There was a sweetness and a humbleness. That's how I knew that he was good and real."

That was twenty years ago, but to look at them their young selves don't seem that far in the past. Bryan is boyish and tan in a baseball cap; his handshake could compress sand into rock. Amanda is pretty with long, loose brunette hair and legs dipped in skinny jeans. You can tell that she's the cool mom. She and Bryan look like they'd have fun on date night.

Except that they never went out to dinner anymore. The stress of caring for a child with a serious medical condition flooded their marriage. The first time they hired a babysitter Hayden was eight. They went to a restaurant down the street, and Amanda called home six times to check in.

Most of the burden fell on Amanda because Bryan, an executive at a global medical device and supply company, had to travel half the month. She was also caring for Hayden's little sister, Ava, and a baby girl named Maggie whom they'd adopted from Guatemala.

For a lot of people, adopting a child on top of managing Hayden's allergies and looking after a second child would have felt like too much. For Amanda and Bryan, it was always part of the plan.

When she was working on her master's degree, Amanda did a clinical rotation at a group home for children awaiting placement in a foster home or adoption. She remembers one day when a family came to pick up a two- and three-year-old. Amanda found two girls, ages nine and eleven, hugging and trying to comfort each other in another room. Because they were older, the girls figured no one was ever going to want to adopt them.

Amanda later told Bryan that someday she wanted to adopt two children in addition to having two of her own. "I'm a very hopeful person and very proactive person," she tells me. She also has a strong Christian faith. "I feel like I've been given so much. This money, this life, is not just for me. This is meant to be shared," she says.

In fact, after Maggie became part of their family, they got pretty far along in the process of adopting a second child from Guatemala when that government shut the system down. For years, Fresh Air Fund kids have spent whole summers at the Hanson house.

Being committed to the children didn't mean that managing all of it didn't flatten her. Finally, Amanda had to let something fall. The something was her husband. By the time the kids were in bed, Amanda was completely tapped out. She had nothing left for Bryan. "There was no capacity left to care for him," she says.

Amanda's single-mindedness and exhaustion are certainly familiar to me. After Shepherd got better, I remember thinking that Darin and I did well as a couple during our ordeal. Looking back, I couldn't remember any fighting. When Darin told me that he'd experienced those months differently, that he thought we were maybe headed for separation, I was shocked.

I realized that the reason I couldn't recall any strain was because

I couldn't recall much about Darin at all from that time. It's really sad for me to think of it now, and incredible, but that's how focused I was on Shepherd. I wouldn't want to draw any conclusions about gender based on two examples, but maybe it's a testament to how overwhelming it is for a mother to have a chronically ill child—and perhaps how strong our biology is; Amanda and I were in survival mode—that we could disregard someone we love that easily. Without even thinking about it.

For Amanda, it would be ten o'clock the night before a birthday party and she would start baking cupcakes and making pizza for Hayden. Bryan would say, "I thought this was time for us." Amanda would respond that he could keep her company in the kitchen or help out if he wanted. He would end up reading or getting on the computer. "It was a complete disconnect," Amanda says.

She was determined to concoct an edible, gluten-free, dairy-free substance that she could pretend was pizza, as well as a cupcake that still qualified as a treat and not a punishment. If she failed, she was sure that Hayden would feel left out of every children's social event since every celebration, regardless of what it claimed to be celebrating, actually celebrated cupcakes and pizza.

Before a birthday party, Amanda would call the mom to find out what she was planning—cake or cupcakes? What color frosting?—so she could try to match it. If you count the birthday celebrations in the classroom and all the parties outside of school, this happened probably thirty times during kindergarten alone. This was on top of shopping and cooking for every meal.

Bryan understood her nurturing impulse, he tells me. But he also felt that she did more than she needed to do. There were baked goods she could have bought at the store. He thought, *You don't need to spend an hour and a half during our time, every time. I get it, but every now and then, let's take the easier path.*

She felt he didn't appreciate all that she did, how wrecked she was, and her bitterness metastasized. Bryan had to travel regularly for business. "'You don't get how serious this is,'" she would say to him. "'You show up for forty-eight hours on the weekend. I've prepped so all the food's ready. To you it looks like no big deal. You try to do this. I should leave for a week. You have no idea how hard it is, emotionally, physically. I can never let my guard down. I'm constantly living under the gun.' I would be crying, but I think he would be like, 'Oh, okay, it can't be that bad,' because he was on the other side of the world."

When she gave up pursuing a career as a therapist to take care of Hayden full-time, she unwittingly got cast as a traditional wife. "God love him," she says of Bryan. "But the reality is—what I've come to terms with is—this is the person I've married. And he is an amazing father, an amazing man. But it's a little bit like a 1950s marriage in some ways. And the thought of that would have once made my skin crawl because I'm not that kind of woman. But somehow, if you really stand back and look at it, we have fallen into these roles. He travels the world. He works. I'm at home with the children."

As much as the allergies flipped over Amanda and Bryan's lives, they took a toll on Hayden, too. Keeping him safe meant making sure everyone knew he was different. His friends kept special drawers full of Hayden-safe snacks for when he came over. At the annual block party he would wear a sign that said PLEASE DON'T FEED ME. It may sound extreme, but having a child with a life-threatening condition pushes you that far.

Like most kids, he didn't want to stand out. He'd always been so-cial, the "walk-up-and-talk-to-you kind," Amanda says. But when he got older, at around seven or eight, he started not wanting to go to parties anymore. "Most birthday parties, you go and you eat. That's a big part of the party," he said to his mom. "What's the point? Don't make the cupcakes anymore," he said. "Don't." Amanda realized that the allergies had scaled her fortress and were starting to damage him. "Oh my gosh," she thought. "He's not in this bubble where I can pro-tect him."

She started thinking ahead. In fifth grade, there was an overnight camping trip. Homecoming. Prom. Everybody goes out to dinner be-fore the dance. What's he going to do? How would he ever go on a date? Or get a job or travel?

He didn't seem anxious—and a large percentage of kids with severe allergies are—but a certain degree of paranoia was unavoidable. At the dinner table he'd ask his mom if she had used his napkin. He'd grab a fresh one to be safe.

Since moving to Colorado, Amanda had stayed in contact with the Boston allergy support group online. It had morphed into a Yahoo! Group that she checked for advice. Somebody posted a question: "Has anybody ever heard of Amy Thieringer?" Amanda thought, *Now, why is that name familiar? I know that name.* And so she tuned in to the back-and-forth. Amy Thieringer, Amanda soon remembered, was the woman with the wand, the one who talked about balancing Hayden's energy to help him tolerate foods that triggered allergy attacks. Some-one wrote, "Oh my doctor said there is no cure for food allergies. That's so risky to try to reintroduce the foods." More people chimed in on that side. But one or two mothers said, "I think we're going to try to start going to her and see if we make any headway." The response was, "Keep us posted on your journey." And then the thread fell silent.

Months went by without another mention of the healer. "I as-sumed it didn't work because it was so quiet," says Amanda.

And then came this post from a mom named Heidi Pasternak, whom Amanda knew from the original support group. "We are having such success with our son, Lucas," she wrote. Amanda remembered liking Heidi, and she remembered that so many of Lucas's allergies were the same as Hayden's and just as severe. So Amanda paid atten-tion every time Heidi would get on to say something. Heidi tells me that she knew it was against the rules of the group, which was moder-ated by a representative from the Asthma and Allergy Foundation of America, to recommend a therapy not based on clinical evidence. But when it seemed clear that Thieringer's therapy was working for Lucas, Heidi felt she had to say something.

Soon Amanda was googling "Amy Thieringer." She found Thiering-er's website, but there was little information about what actually hap-pened in the program. There wasn't a lot to hold on to. This is how it is when you're outside medical science. There can't be a lot of informa-tion because there isn't a lot of information.

Amanda took down the phone number. When she reached

Thieringer, she asked for names and contact information for people whose children had been treated, including Heidi.

Over the phone, Heidi told Amanda about how they were a big Boston Red Sox family, but with Lucas's allergies, they'd been able to go to games only on peanut-free-section nights. Yes, there are peanut-free-section nights. Between 1997 and 2011, the prevalence of food allergies among children seventeen and younger increased from 3.4 to 5.1 percent—a 50 percent jump—according to the Centers for Disease Control and Prevention. Peanut allergies alone more than tripled over roughly the same period among children in the United States, according to a study of self-reported allergies published in *The Journal of Allergy and Clinical Immunology.*

Heidi's family never could have gone to games on other nights. In the closely packed regular stadium seats, you could wind up with peanut dandruff on your shoulders from the guy cracking open shells behind you. It would be easy to inhale a speck of the legume's dust and have a reaction. "If you're a peanut-allergic kid, it's like a death march," Heidi tells me.

Once Lucas's allergies were gone, one of the best things for the family was being able to go to all the games together. "It was the idea that you can exist," Heidi tells me. Heidi emailed Amanda photographic evidence, shots of Lucas posing with a bag of peanuts at the game, his hands cradling his former enemy.

Seafood had been another major threat. Just touching it and licking his finger had been enough to start closing Lucas's throat. "Now Lucas was eating salmon sushi regularly," Amanda tells me. "Like, he's *requesting* it." Amanda talked to two or three more moms. She thought, *That's all the proof I need. This works.* Of course, it wasn't proof in the scientific sense.

Amanda added her name to Thieringer's waiting list, which was six months long at the time, and asked her husband if he could get a transfer to his company's headquarters in Boston. Bryan said it was out of the question; he was now president of the division based in Colorado.

Hayden was seeing a specialist at National Jewish Health in Denver. His doctor initiated a series of challenges, which involved spending the day at the hospital trying increasing amounts of certain foods under close supervision to see if he was still allergic to them. Because blood tests are inconclusive, actually eating the suspect food is the gold standard for determining an allergy.

The doctor chose foods that Hayden had never had a severe reaction to. Hayden actually passed nine of these challenges, but the foods he won back weren't exactly prizes. Canned peas. Kiwi. It was somewhat encouraging, but a life that now allowed for canned peas and kiwi was not a changed life. Hayden still couldn't eat any of the things that were everywhere—gluten-containing grains, dairy, and eggs. The reality was that even though children usually do outgrow certain allergies—to milk, eggs, wheat, and soy—test numbers as high as Hayden's were linked to a decreased likelihood of that happening. Plus, allergies to peanuts, tree nuts, fish, and shellfish, all of which Hayden had, tended to persist.

At the time, though, there was some encouraging news about children with allergies to eggs. Researchers had discovered that a majority of children who were allergic to eggs were able to tolerate them if they'd been baked into a waffle or muffin; heat altered the protein, changing it to a form that no longer provoked an allergic response. Hayden's doctor suggested introducing a baked egg for his next challenge. Amanda thought that getting eggs back would really be something. Her expectations took off.

When Hayden tried the baked egg, though, his lips started swelling. The bad reaction hit Amanda especially hard. For her son to have failed with eggs when so many other kids were having luck with them made the whole food challenge endeavor feel hopeless. It felt like they were getting nowhere.

The conversation Amanda had then with the allergist has stuck with her. She says she told the doctor about the "alternative healer" she was thinking about taking Hayden to. The doctor, Amanda recalls, told her she'd be playing Russian roulette with her child's life. Amanda remembers that it got heated, and that she was crying. When the allergist suggested they come back in six months and try sesame, Amanda thought, *What the fuck is sesame going to do for my kid?* She got up and walked out. The doctor, who was granted permission by Amanda to speak about Hayden's case, declined to comment for this story. According to a written statement from National Jewish Health, Hayden's doctor and primary nurse do not recall discussing an alternative healer with Amanda. It's standard practice to note such conversations, but there's not a mention of it in Hayden's record.

Amanda says that the allergist's disquieting warning followed her out the door. "I remember that put a pit in my stomach," Amanda says. "I walked out of there thinking, 'Am I putting him at risk?'"

But she was resolved. "I remember feeling like, 'They have brought me as far as they could bring me,'" she says. "I knew that it was time to figure something else out." The fact that there were no other established options was not a factor.

How could it not be, though? Most of us would do anything for our children, but Amanda seemed to have a particular fierceness as a mother. She'd had the opposite model in her own father who left his family when Amanda was ten. She wrote him letters afterward, and she never heard back. Amanda would ask her grandmother—his mother—if he'd received them. Yes, she'd tell Amanda, but he has "no comment." This went on for decades. Decades! She was a bright student—straight As—but she was a genius of tenacity. This is what she applied to taking care of her children. If her father took parenting to one extreme, she went as far as she could go the other way. She would do anything for her children and then some—even if it didn't exist yet. It was like mothering on performance-enhancing drugs.

A WEEK LATER THE HANSON family was on vacation in Tucson, Arizona. They'd found a resort that could prepare the right food for Hayden. Amanda had spoken with the chef directly by phone. And it had actually worked out. The whole week they were there, Hayden didn't have any adverse reaction.

Setting out for the twelve-hour drive home, the family stopped at Burger King, one of the few restaurants that served French fries that

Hayden could eat. He ordered a Whopper with nothing on it, not even a bun—a patty with no clothes. Bryan went in, as either he or Amanda always did, to make sure that the meat traveled directly from grill to box. If it ever grazed a bun, they'd ask for a new burger.

Amanda had just passed the bag of food back to the kids. "My throat's feeling really tight, you guys," Hayden said. Under her breath Amanda told Bryan not to get on the highway. Then she launched into her fake-calm voice. "Oh, okay, you're going to be all right. How's it feeling?" They pulled over into a gas station parking lot. Bryan grabbed the GPS to search for a hospital nearby. Amanda kept up her measured performance. "Let's get out of the car, get some fresh air." She asked Hayden, "What are you feeling like?" Bryan was in the car, panicking. The GPS wasn't working; it couldn't find the hospital. The EpiPen was in Amanda's pocket, and she was gripping it.

"It's getting worse, Mom," Hayden was saying. "I think we should go to the hospital." He was doing that swallowing thing. Then Bryan found it. The hospital was a mile and a half away. They jumped back in the car. As they pulled up to the ER doors, Hayden's lips were turning blue.

They got there in time, but Amanda was devastated. *How could this happen again? How could I have not protected him?* she wondered. A sesame seed from a bun must have gotten mixed up in his food, but how? Hayden, as usual, took the situation in stride. He was excited about having his own TV in the hospital and possession of the remote control.

All those years, all those hospital visits, and Hayden never seemed to feel sorry for himself. And sometimes he even felt lucky. One night, when he was seven, and leaving the hospital after yet another anaphylactic reaction, Hayden looked up at the lights on in the windows as they drove away. He said, "I'm so lucky I get to go home tonight. What about all those people who don't get to go home? Someday when I'm older I want to go visit people in hospitals who are sick and talk to them because I know what it feels like." Amanda says, "He's got this old-soul, compassionate quality about him." It's easy to see how his allergies could bloom into empathy.

After several hours in the Tucson hospital, it was safe for Hayden to leave. The Hansons loaded back into their black SUV. The doors clicked shut. Amanda turned to Bryan and said, "I'm moving to Boston."

Six weeks later, a moving truck pulled up outside their Boulder home. Amanda had rented an apartment in Lexington, Massachusetts, without seeing it first because it met her only requirement: It was close to Amy Thieringer's office—six minutes away.

As the movers loaded up some furniture, Bryan started crying. He thought Amanda was risking the family on something he didn't think was going to work. Things had already been not great between them, and now she was going to live across the country. "This is crazy," he told her. "You're going to break our family apart."

"I cannot put my head on the pillow knowing that there's somebody out there who possibly holds the key to our freedom and not try," she told him. "Let me try. After three or four months, if it's not working, I'll come back. I have to try."

And so she effectively became a single mom to her three kids and two dogs. During the first couple of months that they were in Lexington, Amanda also took care of a ten-year-old boy named Naquan, who'd spent the previous three summers staying with the Hansons through the Fresh Air Fund. This summer was no different. Bryan flew in every weekend to be with all of them.

Naturally, Amanda started a blog. She wrote, "It did not matter that my husband's job is in Colorado and he could not go with us. All that did matter were the possibilities for my son's future: Eating in restaurants, freedom to walk onto an airplane without concern of nuts being served, a first kiss without fear the person had eaten something that could kill him." Hayden was now nine years old.

As determined as she was, it was a lot to take on by herself. Hayden's allergies required special attention. And Amanda's daughter Maggie, who was three, also needed a lot of extra care and patience because she had limited language. Just months before the move, the family found out that she was 70 percent deaf.

Amanda had told Thieringer that Hayden's allergies had to be gone in a year; after that, they needed to go back to Colorado. But Thieringer had never worked that fast before and asked if Amanda was sure she wanted to make the move. Thieringer was worried that the stress of Hayden's being away from home would work against his healing.

Amanda was sure.

Amanda and Hayden started seeing Thieringer twice a week. Amy's new office was a sunny space across from the historic Lexington Battle Green. Its design theme could have been called contemporary crayon; it was wallpapered with thank-you cards from children who'd once had severe allergic reactions to certain foods and were now eating everything.

This time, Amanda was ready for whatever Thieringer did. Sure, she was even more desperate. But three and a half years in Boulder, where the streets were paved in granola, had exposed her to the irregular. Plus, she had the testimony of other moms, whom she'd come to trust more than doctors because, she told me, they were the ones in the trenches. It's possible, too, that it was a shoot-the-messenger situation. Doctors didn't have an answer for Hayden's allergies. It wasn't their fault, but Amanda seemed to resent them for it.

As they started their work with Thieringer, Amanda told herself, *This is going to happen.* It was either a thought or a prayer.

It helped that Thieringer's manner inspired confidence. She comes across as extremely self-assured. "I can fix that," she'll say, giving a quick little wave in front of her face as if an allergy were a fly to be swatted.

Thieringer's appearance also goes entirely against type. She wears heels on Saturdays. She has just-came-from-the-salon hair and nails no matter the day. Her skin is tan no matter the month. (The trick, she'll have you know, is to mix self-tanner with lotion, and it won't streak.) She looks astonishingly put together for someone who calls herself a healer. She wears diamonds, not crystals. "We're not burnin' incense, holding hands and singin' some chants," says Amanda. In fact, Thieringer was inclined to say: "Oh my gosh, those are such cute shoes!" The fact that Thieringer was "not a total hippie" made her more credible to Amanda.

Whatever the reason, Amanda connected with her. Although Thieringer still talked about Hayden's energy field, Amanda thought, *This is not some checked-out crazy person.* She tells me, "I think I saw a few of those before."

Amanda and the kids had moved out to Lexington on Memorial Day, so they had a few months there before school started. In the evenings they rode bikes and played in the park. On one of those nights Hayden overheard a mother talking about her daughter's life-threatening food allergies. He asked his mom if he could tell the woman about his energy healer. Hayden grabbed Amy's business card from his mom's purse and scampered over to the woman. From a distance Amanda saw the woman's expression and hurried over.

As Amanda explained the therapy, the woman started laughing and asked if Hayden's doctor approved. Amanda told her she had not gotten permission from her son's doctor. The woman chided Amanda for taking such a risk, warning her, in front of Hayden, that the whole thing would likely backfire. Amanda told her that in eight years of treating children, Thieringer had never had a child go into anaphylaxis. The woman handed back the business card.

When Amanda and Hayden walked away, he grabbed her hand, squeezed it really hard, and said, "I am so happy you are my mom."

By then, Thieringer had been working with Hayden for a couple of months. Her protocol had many components, as mentioned, but the first step was the wand, stylus, and BioScan machine. This was the device that she said registered how quickly electricity completed a circuit through Hayden's body, from stylus to wand, and allowed her to test and see what Hayden was sensitive to.

Thieringer has her clients sit and place their hands on one of those boards with the beanbag underbelly that are made for writing in bed. She sits in a regular office chair, facing the person she's treating. On her laptop she clicks on the name of a substance she wants to test—wheat, lactose, corn, dust, anything. The client holds the wand, and she presses the stylus to his or her finger. A little graph on her computer screen registers the speed of the slight electrical current. She says she can tell, based on the speed, whether the substance is causing a problem or not.

Most of what goes on, however, you can't see. And despite my best efforts, I don't understand how the wand machine works. I can't explain this aspect of the therapy.

Here's what Thieringer says: "You're measuring the flow of energy between two points. You put into that closed circuit a frequency or radio wave which is related to a substance—mold, for example. When I flow the frequency of mold through the circuit, does it go faster or slower? When it flows faster, it means mold is stressing the body."

I know this sounds out there. Untested and obviously strange, it's the kind of thing that journalists like me tend to scoff at. If it hasn't been put through clinical trials and shown to work, then it may as well not exist. But journalists aren't desperate. Parents of sick kids are. When I became one, I no longer had the luxury of dismissing anything. I also realized that there was a difference between knowing that an unproven therapy absolutely did not work and merely lacking evidence that it might.

That said, I still have a hard time with this aspect of Thieringer's therapy. Part of what makes the energy flow scenario so difficult to grasp is that it doesn't correspond to any known biological process. But that's what science is for—deciphering the inexplicable. The scientific method, as we learn in grade school, starts with a hypothesis, a proposed explanation in need of testing. Science always needs different perspectives and new ideas or it couldn't keep moving forward. This therapy—the wand machine plus the many other components of it that Thieringer developed—is certainly a new idea.

In fact, Boston Children's, the Harvard Medical School teaching hospital, is now doing a study testing the efficacy of Thieringer's entire therapy, which she calls Allergy Release Technique. Several Boston Children's patients with severe food allergies had gone to Thieringer and seen good results. One day, Thieringer says, she got a call asking if she'd come in and meet with the allergy group at the hospital. They wanted to hear about her therapy.

The anecdotal evidence is compelling. Through Thieringer, I got in touch with the parents of ninety-four children who all say their kids were helped by the therapy. I also heard back from one adult who was treated herself and said she no longer had allergic reactions, though Thieringer's focus is on children.

Out of that group, the parents of sixty-five children described to me a history of allergic reactions to various foods. They said that after their children underwent Thieringer's Allergy Release Technique, they were able to eat everything without a problem. More than two-thirds of these kids had experienced anaphylaxis previously, in some cases in response to eating tree nuts, peanuts, or shellfish—the allergies that people tend not to outgrow. Everyone has remained tolerant, some going on years. In addition to the sixty-five children who've completed the process, nineteen are still seeing Thieringer; they've become tolerant to some foods but have more to go.

Four people I spoke to quit the therapy even after seeing some success, because their children either wouldn't eat the doses of foods that the process requires, or, in one boy's case, had breathing problems every time he tried to ingest half a peanut, even after successfully eating other foods he'd had allergic reactions to.

Thieringer says that 17 percent of her clients have dropped out before completing the process. Some people get scared off by negative responses, she says. It's also a big commitment and takes time and money; there are those who just aren't willing or able to stick with it, especially if progress stalls or they feel it isn't working, Thieringer says.

The parents of six kids who didn't have traditional food allergies told me about different health issues that resolved after going through the therapy. In most of these cases, the problem was gastritis or eczema, but one mother said that her twelve-year-old daughter had become so debilitated by nausea and fatigue that she quit going to school. When a series of specialists couldn't find any cause, a gastroenterologist diagnosed mental illness. Desperate, her mother called Thieringer, who'd treated the girl's brother for allergies years before. Thieringer suspected the girl was allergic to her braces. She recovered as soon as they were removed.

But, impressive as all this is, there's no objective evidence that the allergies and other issues I heard about didn't subside on their own. I haven't found anyone who is dissatisfied, but because I did not interview everyone Thieringer has ever treated, I don't have enough facts to say what her overall success rate is. This is the kind of helpful information that science, starting with the Boston Children's study, will be able to provide.

Until the entire therapy has been empirically tested, there's no way to know exactly what it's doing, what aspects of it might be having an effect, or what role Thieringer's reassuring manner and the healing environment she fosters play in the results. In the meantime, the Asthma and Allergy Foundation of America, a leading advocacy, education, and research group, doesn't take a position against trying an unsanctioned therapy like Thieringer's. "Medicine is a science and an art," says spokesperson Alex Burgess. "Are there remedies that aren't approved that have helped people? Yes, but AAFA's Medical and Science Council strongly encourages anyone considering unapproved therapies to discuss them with their physicians before beginning therapy."

THIERINGER'S ALLERGY RELEASE TECHNIQUE IS always evolving and involves so many pieces that my description here is not comprehensive. But a core component of it is reintroducing particular foods to the allergic child in ever-increasing doses.

This step is related to oral immunotherapy, which scientists at the major research institutions have been pursuing for years as a possible treatment for allergies. The goal is to desensitize the body to allergens—any substance that induces an allergic response. You start with a tiny, unthreatening amount of food. If the patient can tolerate a teeny bit of it, he or she then graduates to eating a little bit more.

In clinical trials, oral immunotherapy has been somewhat successful in combating allergies. Dr. Wesley Burks, the executive dean of the University of North Carolina School of Medicine, has shown in studies that children who are highly allergic to peanuts can tolerate the life-threatening legume a little at a time. When he started studying oral immunotherapy over a decade ago, it was considered fringe, he tells me. "I had people criticize me a lot about a pretty unconventional treatment. Now twelve years later, there are multiple studies that are showing similar results to the studies we have conducted," he says.

The problem with oral immunotherapy, though, is that no one has been able to prove that it's safe in the long term. A team from Johns Hopkins followed thirty-two children after they underwent oral immunotherapy for milk. Three to five years later, only eight of them were drinking milk without symptoms while nineteen were having reactions, including anaphylaxis. The rest of the group quit drinking milk altogether.

The results of the study, one of the first to look at long-term protection, were discouraging. One of the authors, Dr. Corinne Keet, presented the results to a large, packed room at the 2013 national meeting of the American Academy of Asthma, Allergy & Immunology. "I remember hearing a lot of gasps when I described the subjects continuing to have anaphylaxis in follow-up," Dr. Keet, an associate professor of pediatrics at Johns Hopkins School of Medicine, tells me. "We were especially disappointed that some kids who seemed to do so well at the beginning were having problems."

Though children who continue to consume the problem food regularly after undergoing oral immunotherapy seem to be better protected against an allergic reaction, it is not always the case, Dr. Keet and her Hopkins colleague Dr. Robert Wood write in their 2014 review in *The Journal of Clinical Investigation*. At this point there's no clear way to predict who will lose their tolerance down the road and have a potentially deadly reaction. The odds of a fatality, however, are probably very low, Dr. Keet tells me.

On the more positive side, other studies have shown that when the desensitization process lasts for a longer period of time—for three or four years, compared to one year in the Hopkins study—the tolerance seems to stick better. Trials continue, but the early excitement about oral immunotherapy as a possible cure for allergies has faded somewhat. It has not been approved by the Food and Drug Administration (FDA).

MIND OVER PEANUTS

Thieringer's Allergy Release Technique was based on the idea that oral immunotherapy wasn't enough. Desensitization was an important part, but she felt that before you could begin to reintroduce a food to an allergic child like Hayden, you first needed to treat his fear.

When you're taught that something can kill you, you learn to be afraid. It's basic survival. Thieringer believed that Hayden's fear of certain foods was then reinforced over years of ambulance rides, ER visits, absorbing his parents' panic. Some of the symptoms of anaphylaxis—nausea, rapid heart rate, dizziness, fainting—can look an awful lot like a panic attack.

Seeing a connection between anxiety and allergies, Thieringer believed she had to defuse the emotion before she could head off an attack. In her view, allergies were as much a psychological issue as a physiological one.

The idea was that by ratcheting down Hayden's fear of certain foods, his overactive immune system would also become calm. If you could relieve the stress, her thinking went, the immune cells would become less likely to overreact in an allergic reaction.

In an effort to bring down Hayden's anxiety—to try to change how he regarded certain foods that he'd spent a lifetime being afraid of—Thieringer used ideas from cognitive behavioral therapy, a common form of psychotherapy. There's good evidence that cognitive behavioral therapy, or CBT, can be an effective way to treat anxiety. Even so, it was quite a leap to use it as part of a treatment for allergies. CBT doesn't cure anxiety; rather, it helps a person be aware of worries when they start to infiltrate his or her mind—and to take a critical look at them.

One of the things anxiety does to us is distort situations, making them seem much worse than they are. CBT teaches a person to pause and examine stressful events clearly, noticing any inaccurate, exaggerated, or negative thoughts: to step outside the vortex of fear and avoid being swept up in a panic.

All the same, cognitive therapy recognizes that anxiety is a haunted house that you sometimes can't avoid entering, as a therapist once described it to me. Once you're inside, it helps your overall nervous state to know that the ghosts are fake. This is what CBT trains a person to do—to recognize that the white sheets are costumes.

With Hayden, Thieringer's use of CBT concepts was as straightforward as telling him that in those moments of worrying about what eating the wrong food could do to him, he needed to remind himself that he was strong and safe. To drive the point home, Thieringer suggested he repeat the mantra: "My allergies are gone. I can eat anything." Even though it was not exactly the case that his allergies were gone, saying something like "I'm learning to tolerate foods again" didn't have the same punch. He also needed to remember that if he did have a reaction, he could always use an EpiPen, take antihistamines, or drink Alka-Seltzer Gold tablets dissolved in water—oddly enough, Alka-Seltzer Gold is thought to calm down allergic processes.

The wand machine was supposed to be an evaluation tool, but it was also something of an acupuncture device. Remember the energy pathways that Thieringer said she was tapping into with the stylus that emitted an electrical circuit? In traditional Chinese medicine, those pathways are called meridians, and blockages in them are seen as being linked to disease. Though scientists use different language to describe it than Thieringer does, they have shown that stimulating acupuncture points, which is what she seemed to be doing with her current of electricity, causes the brain to release endorphins, those soothing pain-conquering hormones, according to a 2008 review in *The Journal of Alternative and Complementary Medicine*. A group at Harvard Medical School using functional MRI (fMRI)—imaging that maps and measures brain activity—showed that when acupuncture points were stimulated, areas of the brain associated with fear quieted down, according to a 2005 article in *Human Brain Mapping*. This could possibly explain how Thieringer's machine might mollify Hayden's stress—and prepare him to try certain foods again.

When I ask UNC's Dr. Burks, the oral immunotherapy pioneer, about acupuncture, he tells me that he thinks it's possible that the ancient practice could have a role in how we respond to an allergen or how we perceive the symptoms that we have from allergies or treatment. "Our mind and body interact," he says. "It's not like they're just two separate processes independent of each other." Science, as we'll learn later, is starting to understand this relationship better.

Along the same lines, Hayden was also taught to tap acupressure points on his face and chest—to gently thump his fingertips to his temples and chin, for example—while he said the reassuring words of his mantra: "My allergies are gone. I can eat anything."

This combination of acupressure point stimulation and concentration on a particular issue was also thought to calm fear. It was a variation of a therapy developed by the psychologist Roger Callahan. Though the practice is not mainstream, a 2012 review of eighteen randomized, controlled trials of acupressure point stimulation—through tapping, massage, or pressure—combined with the mental exercise suggests that it has a strong positive effect on various psychological disorders including post-traumatic stress disorder (PTSD), phobias, and anxiety. How it worked was a mystery, but the authors, writing in *Review of General Psychology,* speculated that the tapping may act on the brain as the needles of acupuncture seem to, by calming fear centers.

Thieringer also did tapping herself, lightly rapping her knuckles up and down Hayden's vertebrae, a practice she borrowed from Reiki. (She is a certified Reiki master.) Originating in Japan, Reiki is described as an energy therapy intended to create a sense of peace and calm through touch, though it has not been rigorously studied, according to the NIH's National Center for Complementary and Integrative Health.

Thieringer's tapping—like the stimulation of acupuncture points—conceivably sent signals up Hayden's spine, resulting in an endorphin rush.

Thieringer was constantly working to change the way Hayden thought about food and his body's reaction to it. She explained to him that his overactive immune cells were trying to protect him, like fire-fighters. They just overdid it. Hayden needed to tell his amped-up immune cells, "Thanks, but no thanks"—to send the firefighters back to the station.

Sometimes, Thieringer tapped into Hayden's subconscious, she said, to communicate that food was his friend, not an enemy. This in-volved saying the words to herself.

Amanda rolled with it. She was all in at this point. She didn't feel she had to understand exactly what Thieringer was doing or why. It wasn't hurting Hayden, and maybe it would help him, as it had helped others.

The campaign to ease Hayden's fear of the foods he was allergic to continued at home. Under Thieringer's direction, Amanda and the four kids made posters of all the things Hayden would soon be able to eat. They listed the ways his life would improve, starting with being able to order anything off the ice cream truck. They hung the posters next to a big calendar where they marked off the days until they could all go home to Colorado.

Again, there was no empirical evidence that all of this would free Hayden from his allergies. But Amanda and her children were there in Lexington, after all, because they'd tapped out medicine and sci-ence.

What did Hayden make of his sessions with Thieringer? "The first time it was weird, but then it got normal," he told me later, when he was twelve.

AFTER ABOUT SIX WEEKS OF running electrical currents, working to correct Hayden's fear of certain foods, and lots of tapping, Thieringer said he was ready to try a hard-boiled egg. She put a speck of it on his hand. The next time she saw him, she dabbed it on his chin, then below his lip, then on his lip. Amanda was so impatient to get on with it already, she wasn't even nervous when Hayden finally got to lick the squishy yellow dot off his lip.

He didn't love the taste, honestly, but unlike the last time he'd tried a cooked egg, before he'd begun working with Thieringer, his body didn't react.

This was progress.

As his doses of the hard-boiled egg increased, Thieringer continued to lull him with the idea that it was all okay, using her rainbow of tools—the wand machine, the ideas from CBT, the tapping—to keep his body calm. Then she introduced dairy.

As willfully confident as Amanda had been that the therapy would work, her son's new tolerance was still stunning to witness. "As sure as I am typing this," she wrote on her blog, "I saw with my own two eyes my son lick dairy off of [his lip] yesterday & today without any reaction. Tomorrow we up the daily dose & by his birthday in November he will have a scoop of ice cream in a bowl. Something he has NEVER experienced!"

Bryan quickly got on board. But that didn't make the distance any easier to bridge. Naquan, from the Fresh Air Fund, left at the end of summer, but Amanda was still caring for a little girl with special needs, her daughter Maggie, and getting Hayden through his therapy. And they were living away from home. Handling just one of those would have been plenty, even for someone with Amanda's mothering gusto, drive, and independence. If she was spent before, now Amanda was so worn out it was easier not to fill Bryan in on their days. "The word 'the' was too much," she says.

As her daughter Maggie struggled to communicate, she did a lot of hitting and yelling. "I think there was guilt that I should have been working with her even more than I was because I was so consumed with working with Hayden," Amanda says. "I remember feeling so exhausted after dinner and thinking, 'I have to read to this child.' That's what they kept saying, 'You cannot read enough to her.' So even if I read her five books, I'd feel like I should have read ten. I was going to bed feeling like no matter what I did it wasn't enough."

Thieringer told Amanda that it was important to have a serene environment while Hayden was eating his servings of the various foods he was working on. Amanda leaned on Ava, then seven, for help. She'd ask Ava to take Maggie upstairs and let her play with her Barbies for twenty minutes. "Here are some cookies. I'll let you stay up ten extra minutes."

Between visits to Thieringer, Hayden worked on the food desensitization at home. As he worked his way up to tolerating larger amounts of certain foods, he would sometimes have a physical response to them. He and his mom had a scale from one to ten that tracked anything Hayden might be feeling, ten being trouble breathing. Early on in the process he had some occasional tingling and itching after increasing a dose, but it always resolved quickly after he tapped acupressure points on his face (really), repeated his mantra (really), and drank an Alka-Seltzer Gold dissolved in water (really).

One afternoon, after upping his serving of oyster crackers, a step toward tolerating wheat, Hayden said, "Mom, I'm at a four. Actually a five." Amanda said, "Oh, that's okay. Let's do our tapping and take an Alka-Seltzer Gold. This is just your body processing through the wheat."

"Mom, I do not feel well, I'm at a seven now."

"No worries. You are just fine. Finish your Alka-Seltzer."

"Mom, I can't swallow it. We need to go to the hospital."

At this point Amanda felt around behind her back for the EpiPen she kept in the pencil jar on the counter. She was secretly taking the cap off, trying to project calm. At that moment, Ava came in the room, saw Hayden's face, and started screaming, "OMG, are we going to the hospital? Is Hayden having trouble breathing?"

Hayden started to tremble and whimper and Amanda finally chucked the acting routine. "You either finish that Alka-Seltzer or I have to EpiPen you right now!" She'd never seen him chug anything so fast. Twenty seconds passed. Hayden looked at his mom and started to smile. "I'm at a one, Mom. I'm going to be okay." A couple of minutes later, he asked if they could have lunch soon. He was starving.

❀   ❀   ❀

AMANDA WAS NEARING THE LIMIT of what she could handle, and she aimed her frustration at Bryan. As Amanda tells it, "He'd say, 'You think you're the only one going through this. We're all going through this. I'm not with you guys.' I'm like, 'I get it. I do. But you're still flying on the corporate jet. You're still staying at five-star hotels all over the world, having beautiful dinners and bottles of wine. It's a little bit different.'"

That fall, having vanquished some threats but still vulnerable to quite a few more foods, Hayden got strep and his body started rejecting the new doses of food. Thieringer suggested holding off on moving forward for a while. Amanda wondered how they'd ever make it home in a year, by the next Memorial Day. At the same time she found out that she needed surgery on her wrist and wouldn't be able to drive. "I'd never had a hint of depression my entire life," says Amanda. "But I remember bawling, in the fetal position on the couch." She told Bryan she couldn't do it anymore. Could he please come out for two weeks to help. Bryan said he wasn't able to. She told him, "If this was cancer, you would be on the plane. Food allergies could kill him. It's just as serious. I'm begging you. I need you right now." And still he told her, "I can't do that," according to Amanda.

Bryan remembers it a little differently. Because he had a board meeting he couldn't miss, he asked Amanda if her mom might be able to fly in for the two weeks after her surgery. It turned out that she was available to help out. If Amanda's mom hadn't been able to come, Bryan says, "I never would have left her in a situation like that." They didn't talk about alternatives, but maybe Bryan would have asked his own mom, Amanda says.

Amanda took a black-and-white view, accusing him of prioritizing his job over her, he says. They were lucky that Bryan was successful enough to cover two households and the out-of-pocket expense of the therapy. As in other stories in this book, having enough money to try iffy things was no small detail. Insurance doesn't cover unsanctioned therapies. The fact was, Bryan did have to make sure work went well; everything depended on it.

Amanda didn't seem to be aware that the year was tough on him, too. He already felt awful that he wasn't able to be there during the week, but Bryan says Amanda lumped on more guilt. He says the message he got from her was: "'You're just not doing enough, and I'm suffering.'" He tells me, "It was almost like it was my fault."

He flew across the country every weekend to be with them, landing at one a.m. on a Friday, which was plenty grueling. The effort didn't register. "I justified it in my mind that it was really, really hard for her," he says. "You can't help being a bit self-centered at that time. That's the way I got through it, trying to put myself in her position. It would have been great to have someone say, 'I know this is hard for you, too.' But I don't blame her for it."

It hurts him more in reflection, he tells me. "You're not in the middle of the war now, so maybe you can rethink it." But the way that she tells the story is that he didn't do anything. "It still feels now that it wasn't a shared experience," he says.

After Amanda pleaded with Bryan to come out for those two weeks and he didn't, her resentment swelled as if it were its own allergic response. She felt that his attitude was, "It's your thing. You made the decision. Don't call me crying about how hard this is. Do it and deal with it."

Even though they found help for Amanda after her wrist surgery, what she really needed had less to do with logistics. Bryan thought he'd found a solution by suggesting her mom; to Amanda, it registered as a betrayal because what she was really asking for was emotional support, the kind that could only come from him. "It's that feeling, and even talking about it now I could almost cry. It just brings up that feeling of: There's really nobody to lean on."

When Amanda's father left her family, there was no one else she felt she could fall back on then, either. Her mother remarried. At sixteen, Amanda asked her grandmother if she could move in with her. The grandmother, who was in her eighties, was struggling financially.

She told Amanda that she could live there but that she'd have to help pay the bills. Amanda got two jobs and left her mom's house.

One night, after Amanda had worked late closing the yogurt shop where she worked, the old Buick Regal she'd bought with her own money died halfway to home. Her first worry was that she had so much homework to do. She walked along a dark street to a pay phone and called her mother, but she wasn't home. Her grandmother didn't have a car. She didn't think she could call any of her girlfriends at that hour. Amanda had to think, who am I going to call? She thought of her dad. "I remember thinking it was such a desperate move," she says now. Her father picked up and told her, "We're just getting ready for bed. Can you call someone else?"

There was one other person, a boyfriend that she'd recently broken up with. He came to get her.

When the filament between Amanda and Bryan finally gave way, she quickly found her footing. "You can't come? Mm-kay. Then I will do this by myself," she thought. Self-reliance, after all, was her habit. As it so often is with patterns that originate in childhood, slipping back into solo mode for Amanda was seamless. This was her natural state.

She began construction on a wall that blocked Bryan out. *I'm in this court with my little people and you're over there,* she thought to herself. They continued to talk on the phone, but Amanda kept simmering, often letting his calls go to voicemail. She didn't consider going home to Colorado.

After a few weeks off, Hayden started up his work with Thieringer again, and this time his body was game. They progressed quickly through more allergens, the foods that had provoked an allergic reaction before.

When they arrived in late May, Hayden avoided dairy, wheat, rye, barley, eggs, sesame, peanuts, and tree nuts. Eight months later he was scarfing down almost everything. In one three-week span he had his first doughnut, pizza, bagel, peanut, scone, breadstick, onion ring, and hamburger bun, which was sesame to boot.

Amanda wrote on her blog, "YES! YES! YES! IT IS WORK-ING!!!!!!! WE ARE DOING IT!!!!!"

Hayden, who by then was ten, told Amanda, "Mom, it's like I have landed on Mars. It's all so strange and exciting at the same time. Every time I taste new foods my taste buds are overwhelmed and then I realize I like it and I want more."

One night, the family went out to an Asian-fusion restaurant. Hayden was eating so quickly, Amanda reminded him to chew his food and to breathe. "But Mom," he said, "I've waited ten years for this."

They made their deadline of knocking out all of Hayden's allergies in a year. They'd done it. She'd solved a huge family problem. "I think I felt super-victorious. I felt super-relieved. And I never felt closer to my kids," she says. She'd lived up to words she'd used on them again and again: to trust their instincts. The experience affected how she felt about herself. "I feel like something shifted in me as a mother, in my second-guessing of myself." Now, she says about her instincts as a parent, "I'm really sure."

Once she and the kids were back in Colorado, she was practically manic. One afternoon right after their return Hayden went out to play with some buddies on the local soccer fields. Amanda went by after a while to see if any of them were hungry. She ended up ordering three large pizzas for five children. Another mom gawked at Hayden as he dug in. "Are you sure this is okay?" she said. In fact, Thieringer insists that her clients keep eating all the foods they've mastered in order to maintain tolerance.

Once the family was back together again in Colorado, there was still one thing that needed to be fixed. Amanda and Bryan had gone in two different directions. Now that she was home, it was clear just how far. And the physical separation wasn't over. Two weeks after her return Bryan was promoted again, this time to a position in Connecticut. If Amanda had waited a year to start working with Thieringer, her move to Lexington would not have been necessary. At this point Amanda felt so disconnected from Bryan that she didn't go with him to the East Coast. "I would just as soon have him gone," she thought then. "He can go do his thing. I'll do my thing." It would be a full year before she and the kids would join him.

Bryan, though, persevered. *No matter how bad it gets, we're married,* he thought. *We'll figure it out.* They started counseling during his visits back to Colorado. In therapy together, Amanda talked about feeling abandoned by Bryan, which had dredged up old pain from her childhood, her father's exit. "No amount of yoga can cure that wound," she tells me. She realized that she'd been pinning all of that history on Bryan.

For the first time, she says, she understood that the year had been rough on Bryan, too. He got emotional explaining how he didn't have the choice to be able to help her in Lexington. That year, he was either working or flying, which created extraordinary stress that he didn't feel he could ever share with her. There wasn't room for anyone else's problems but hers; he had to be the strong one. And when he visited, he felt like an outsider in his own family because Amanda and the kids were in their own groove. "I didn't realize until therapy how hurt he was," Amanda tells me.

It helped to talk. They also started hiring babysitters regularly and going out to dinner. Applying the doggedness they'd practiced the year before, they said, "My God, we went through all of that. We can't fall apart now."

After joining Bryan in Connecticut, Amanda became the Fresh Air Fund's representative in Fairfield and helped found Believe Guatemala, an organization that offers counseling, tutoring, and funding for private school tuition to families in Guatemala City. She and Bryan never gave up their plan to adopt two children on top of having two of their own. In 2016, they became the legal guardians of Naquan, now seventeen, who'd continued to spend every summer with the family.

Amanda's years studying psychology didn't go to waste. Her children and their friends are often hanging out in the kitchen. She credits her schooling with knowing how to relate to them, making them comfortable. I ask her if she thinks her psychology background played a role in how she dealt with Hayden's allergies. "Not as much as my personality," she says.

Though the family has moved on, part of Amanda misses the intensity of those allergy years, like a soldier home from war. "As crazy as that sounds—there was something about the focus of being in the fight," she says. "The closeness."

At first Bryan and Amanda thought they'd hold on to the EpiPens, just in case. But the film of worry washed away. When I meet him a couple of years later, Hayden remembers that it was pretty scary whenever his throat would close. But he never thinks about it anymore, he tells me.

That's how it feels when you're free.

HAYDEN TURNED SIXTEEN IN 2016. He's quick with a smile and a handshake. He plays hockey. He's taller than his mom. And, in the six years since he graduated from Thieringer's program, he hasn't had a single bad reaction to food.

He hangs out in a close group of friends. A while ago, though, Amanda noticed that he'd stopped going to parties. She asked him why, and he just said he didn't feel like it. Then two weeks later he went to her and told her that some kids had started smoking marijuana. He'd been offered it and said no, but he felt enormous pressure. Amanda asked him why he'd refused. His bottom lip started trembling. He couldn't answer her right away. He looked like the five-year-old boy he'd once been.

Then he pointed at her and finally said, "Because of you." Amanda looked at him. He said, "Because of all those years ago when you worked so hard to get my body healthy. I don't want to do anything to mess that up."

8

Jamie Stelter

The Raw Fuel of Optimism

*If you tell me it's not going to kill me, I will try it. I might even try
something if you told me it might kill me if it will make me feel better.*
—JAMIE STELTER

JAMIE STELTER, A TV REPORTER, WAS AT WORK THE DAY BEFORE
Halloween in 2014 when she got the email she'd been waiting patiently for—or *not* so patiently. She'd been checking her account in
between takes on air. She delivered traffic and transit news to viewers
of the cable news channel New York 1 six times an hour, from five to
nine-thirty in the morning. She had arrived that day for work at her
usual four a.m. She was like the army, doing more before nine a.m.
than most of us did all day.

Her mom, Helen Shupak, was always the first person she heard
from. She tuned in every morning at five to see her daughter. After
Jamie's first spot Helen would send her a text message, usually telling
her how pretty she looked.

Jamie was edgy this morning. As she kept an eye on her in-box, she roused her Twitter account and set it loose to do the thing it did best—devour the minutes. She tweeted that frozen pears lent a "luxe" texture to a smoothie. She tweeted that the F train was in business again after an earlier diversion onto the G line. Finally, that critical email showed up. It was a notification from the doorman of her apartment building letting her know that she had a package at the front desk.

Once she heard that the package had arrived, she wasn't about to stick around. Despite the urgency, she couldn't hurry. For months, her right ankle had been too painful to bend. She limped out of NY1's studio in Chelsea to catch a cab. "I was dragging my foot behind me," she says.

Her ankle started bothering her a year before. She had rheumatoid arthritis, so it wasn't the first time she'd felt pain in a joint, but it was the first time one involved in walking was giving her trouble.

Jamie lives in a loft building in Manhattan's West Village. Stepping up to the front desk where the deliveries were kept, she greeted the doorman, her good cheer booming through the lobby. In this respect the day was no different from any other. She was always extravagant with warmth.

The doorman handed over a huge box. She hefted it onto one shoulder of her petite, five-foot-one frame and hobbled over to the elevator bank, her cargo swaying above her. She'd paid $1,000 for this bundle. (Shipping alone was $100.)

Inside the box were two large plastic bags filled with dry ice. Underneath the ice was one brown paper lunch bag. Inside that bag was a small white plastic bottle. Inside the bottle were forty capsules. And Russian-dolled inside those capsules were other capsules. And inside those capsules was poop.

THE PAIN IN JAMIE'S JOINTS started when she was twenty-one years old. She was home from college for winter break. She kept waking up with swollen, painful hands. "Oh my God!" she says now with customary zest. "They were red, giant basketballs inside my knuckles."

Her mom took Jamie to see a pediatrician, who referred her to a rheumatologist. That doctor drained the fluid from her knuckles before she went back to school for her last semester at the University of Maryland. The relief was temporary. By the time she graduated and was back home for the summer, she could no longer button her own pants. Opening jars was also out.

The pain was especially bad in her knuckles. She'd never realized how much she relied on that particular joint—such a tiny piece of equipment—until it was kaput. "It rendered your whole hand useless," she says.

It didn't occur to her that she had a disease. "I was such a healthy person," she says. "Those things don't happen to healthy, young, skinny people." She figured she was having a reaction to something. She thought, *They're going to give me medicine, and I'll be better.* In the meantime, she just worked around her new difficulties. *I guess I won't have the peanut butter today because I can't open the jar,* she would say to herself.

Her plan was to get a job as a TV news reporter. She'd figured out early that she wanted to be in front of an audience. She tried gymnastics, then singing—she was constantly auditioning for solos in the synagogue choir. The only problem was that she had a terrible voice.

In seventh grade, for a project about the Olympics, she had her dad videotape her doing fake newscasts around town, pretending she was reporting from various athletic events. She took several outfits to change into. She realized that being a TV news reporter was her ticket to the stage. She was twelve years old, and from that point on she would tell people that someday she was going to be on TV.

You would have been a fool to think she wouldn't get what she wanted, as Jamie's eighth-grade American history teacher learned. He offered his students an opportunity for extra credit that for some reason she missed. She kept bothering her teacher about getting another chance, to the point where her parents told her to leave him alone. She didn't. Finally she came up with her own extra credit—on spec. She told her teacher that she had memorized all of the American presidents in a song that she'd made up. He told her, fine, she'd get the extra credit if she sang the song in front of the class. "I still know the song now. If I was in a pageant, that would be my trick," she says. "My parents are always like, 'You need to calm down.'"

But Jamie just wasn't built that way. Perennially effervescent, she lived on the bright side, always making molehills out of mountains. "No one was ever going to tell me that I couldn't do something," she says. "Ever."

The summer after college, while waitressing, she made a dozen copies of her reel, a VHS tape compiling all the fake stand-ups she'd done while interning at TV stations during college. She sent the tapes to stations all over the country.

And she kept seeing doctors about her hands. Finally, after three months, she got the RA diagnosis.

To treat the painful inflammation in her fingers, the doctor prescribed prednisone, a steroid, and methotrexate, the same highly effective immune suppressant my son Shepherd took. Her hands felt better almost immediately. *Well this is fine,* she thought. *I can just take these.* She was focused on just wiping out the pain. "It wasn't like, 'What's in this drug? What is this drug doing to my body?'" she tells me. "It was just like, 'My fucking hands hurt. Let's stop this.'"

Right before Thanksgiving she heard from News 12 Long Island. They liked her tape, they told her, and they needed a traffic reporter. She told them she wanted to be a news reporter, and she didn't know any roads. They told her they'd teach her traffic and would eventually let her do hard news, but right then they needed a traffic reporter and they wanted her. She knew she could have ended up anywhere. "So I was like, 'Fuck! Long Island instead of Kansas? I'm there!'"

During her first two years on the job in Long Island, she continued to take the prednisone and methotrexate, but over time she needed to up her doses to control the soreness in her fingers. While she fended off the inflammation in her hands, she was losing the battle on a new front. Her wrists, too, had been land-grabbed by tenderness and pain. She also noticed she always felt tired, but it was hard to say whether this was the RA, her medication, or her new early schedule.

In 2004, Jamie started seeing a new rheumatologist who gave her repeated cortisone injections in her wrists to take away the pain. "I still was thinking at the time, 'I'm going to go back to being fine.'" Her mom, Helen, was similarly confident. "Who would have ever thought that it was lifelong, that it would always be in her body?" Helen tells me.

It now sounds quaint that neither of them did their own research about RA. It wasn't that long ago, but it seems like a completely different time in terms of information and medicine. Those were the days before googling a disease—or anything—was a reflex, when we depended on doctors for our health information. Jamie's doctors must not have shared the cruel fact that RA didn't go away or that she'd likely be on medication for life.

Today there are worries about frequent use of cortisone because over time it can eat away at the joint it's meant to protect. Jamie was getting multiple injections per visit and would go back for more every couple of weeks because the cortisone brought such relief. She never questioned her doctor, she says, because she "felt like superwoman after an injection." This went on for several years.

By the time she was twenty-five she could no longer bend her wrists. Years of sustained inflammation, despite treatment, had ground down the substance of the joints, narrowing the distance between the bones to such an extent that there was no room to move. The cortisone shots could also have contributed to the erosion of the cartilage there. Even so, the rheumatologist Jamie began to see in 2007, Dr. Harry D. Fischer, chief of the division of rheumatology at Mount Sinai Beth Israel in New York, attributes the loss of use to the progression of Jamie's disease. "This is what rheumatoid arthritis does," says Dr. Fischer, who spoke to me with Jamie's permission.

The only upside was that she no longer felt arthritis pain there because the wrist joints were essentially eliminated.

Meanwhile, the medication had reached a stalemate against the inflammation in her fingers. Most days she was able to use them okay, but more severe soreness would come and go with her period, the rain, a bad night's sleep. Even though her fingers didn't ever feel great, they felt much worse whenever she tried to lower her doses of medication.

Whatever pain she had was now accompanied by a general feeling of weakness, in addition to the old fatigue. At the Long Island TV station, getting ready to go on air every morning was physically difficult for her. It was an hour-long ordeal that usually started with muscling on Spanx. She did her own hair, which required holding a round brush and blow-dryer over her head for an extended period. Her dark brown hair was long—it took forever to dry. Then she'd go through the whole thing with a curling iron. Like any set of tools, these required dexterity and strength. But some days she could barely lift her arms, and she was never able to grip anything that well. "Even doing my makeup. It doesn't sound like a lot, but when your arms and your hands hurt, it's a lot." She loved her job, but on bad days the prep work was so daunting that she started to think about finding another career.

In the late '90s a new class of RA drugs, called biologics, came on the market. They target the parts of the immune system that trigger inflammation. Rheumatologists say the drugs have revolutionized the treatment of RA, but they come with an increased risk of infection, as well as lymphomas and other tumors. Jamie tried both of the blockbusters, Humira and Enbrel. Her boyfriend at the time helped with the injections the drugs required. Each one seemed to work initially, but the effect never lasted.

As with so many diseases, finding a therapy that works for RA is often trial and error. When X-rays showed a severe narrowing of the spaces between the joints in her fingers—a threat to her continued ability to use them—Dr. Fischer was concerned. The change had occurred over a single year. He told Jamie she could try a new biologic medication or an infusion of a drug called Rituxan, which is a chemotherapy used to treat certain types of non-Hodgkin's lymphoma. It can also be effective in blocking the part of the immune system that attacks joints in people with RA, particularly those who, like Jamie, have had little luck with other drug therapies.

Jamie went for the Rituxan. Helen came up from Pennsylvania on the train to be with her daughter during the treatment. At the hospital, she got off the elevator and realized Jamie had sent her to the cancer floor. She felt sick to her stomach. "What didn't she tell me? She didn't tell me! This is how she's going to tell me?" says Helen. "It was like such . . . you know how . . . just your heart . . ."

Helen found Jamie in the chemotherapy room, its walls painted illness beige. A tube octopused from a bag of fluid into her daughter's arm, but Jamie quickly assured her mother that she did not have cancer. As the two passed the hours chatting and flipping through magazines, Helen pretended she wasn't freaked out to be there with her daughter.

Jamie wasn't rattled by the idea of getting chemotherapy because she was focused on the new chance at success, a buoyancy that would come to define how she approached her disease, as it did the way she went through life. "If you tell me it's not going to kill me, I will try it. I might even try something if you told me it might kill me if it will make me feel better."

Rituxan actually *can* kill you. The risk to RA patients is extremely rare—eight times less likely than getting struck by lightning, says Dr. Fischer. But some people who have received it have developed progressive multifocal leukoencephalopathy, or PML, which is an uncommon infection of the brain that cannot be treated, prevented, or cured and that usually causes death or severe disability, according to a National Institutes of Health warning.

Jamie doesn't remember being told about PML, but Dr. Fischer reads to me a note from her file: "Risks discussed in detail." He also says she let him know in an email that she'd done her own research on Rituxan. Anyway, as she said, she was all for anything that might make her better, regardless of the possibility of negative consequences.

PRETTY SOON AFTER THE INFUSION Jamie was in pain, so it was not something she tried again. It had been four years since her diagnosis, and she finally understood that her situation was serious. Her boyfriend could be startlingly frank about it. Jamie says, "I would always talk about how I wanted to have all these kids, and everybody handles these things differently, but he would be like, 'How are you going to have kids? You can't open a spaghetti jar?' It sort of sank in to me at that point.

"I would be so upset, of course, but he was watching me get worse and anything you read tells you, this is a debilitating disease. And, sure, his bedside manner was terrible, but he wasn't wrong for the fears he was having," she says. Her boyfriend tells me in an email that he never gave up hope that they could have children. "We were best friends and lovers so we said a lot of things to each other. [But] I never said it like you have in your quote."

It was through her boyfriend that Jamie was first introduced to other potential therapies for her arthritis. She'd meet him at his office after work and end up chatting with his boss. One day, the boss told her about his tennis elbow and the holistic treatments he'd had success with. He was the first person to suggest to her that drugs weren't the only option.

After that conversation Jamie started to wonder about what she was taking. She thought, "I'm taking all these medications, and I still don't feel great. If I'm gonna take all of those, I should feel awesome. But the medicine just dulled everything and made it so I could manage life and feel okay. It was never solved."

Now she wanted to solve it.

Because onward was her default setting, she simply brushed by the fact that there was no known cure for RA. She went to see the boss's Chinese acupuncturist and felt complete relief from the pain constantly lurking in her joints. As with the medicines she tried, though, the effect didn't last. She felt like whatever the acupuncture was doing, it wasn't getting to the root of her problem.

The acupuncturist had recommended she give up meat and dairy, but she didn't see how that was going to help her. But then, after a particularly painful evening—she and her boyfriend had gone to New Orleans to celebrate her birthday with friends, and she ended up retreating to her hotel room—she woke up and reached for the acupuncturist's advice about what to eat. She had to keep trying—something, anything—and this was the last crumb in her cabinet of ideas.

They flew home the next day and she emptied her kitchen. She bought new groceries at a place called, untantalizingly, Integral Yoga Natural Foods. "At the time it wasn't like you could get organic or vegan food or gluten-free everywhere," she says. It was 2007. "It wasn't how it is now."

"I went vegan and literally three days later I am making a full, strong fist and punching my boyfriend in the arm," she says. "It cured me."

It sure seemed like it had.

Jamie was a true believer in the power of her new diet. "I buy Alicia Silverstone's *The Kind Diet*," she says of the actress's vegan cookbook. "And it became my bible. I made every food in there. And I studied every word." Jamie tried things she'd never heard of before, like umeboshi, which are pickled plums. She was big on making the chocolate peanut butter cups for dinner parties, to show people that vegan desserts were delicious, too. And quinoa. "We ate a lot of quinoa back then," she says.

Like most rheumatologists, Dr. Fischer didn't have much to say about diet. "Jamie's very proactive in her treatment and certainly there are things that can't hurt her as far as I know," he tells me. "And certainly if they provide benefits, I think that's, you know," he says.

And yet, there is some evidence that particular diets can have an effect on RA symptoms. These studies come with the usual caveat, however, that diet can't be studied as rigorously as drugs because it's difficult to blind people to what they're eating.

In a study published in the highly respected British medical journal *The Lancet* in 1991, twenty-seven rheumatoid arthritis sufferers were isolated on a "health farm" and, following a week of fasting, were fed a gluten-free, vegan diet that was individually adjusted—meaning that if someone noticed any increase in symptoms following the reintroduction of a food, it would be omitted from his or her diet. The control group ate a regular diet at a convalescent home. After four weeks, the researchers measured grip strength, how long the participants felt stiff in the morning, how many joints were swollen and tender, and several markers of inflammation in the blood. The people on the special diet showed "significant improvement" compared with those who ate normally. (Both groups reported less pain.) Over the next year, the diet group was gradually reintroduced to gluten and dairy but kept eating those foods only if their arthritis didn't get worse. At the end of the twelve months, they'd held on to all their gains.

In a 2003 study in *Annals of Rheumatoid Diseases,* twenty-six Swedes with RA followed a Mediterranean diet, which includes a lot of fish, olive oil, fruits, vegetables, and legumes, for twelve weeks. Along with free bottles of olive oil, they also got an improvement in inflammatory activity and physical function, among other factors, without changing their dose of medication. The people in the control group suffered in two ways—they didn't feel better and they were fed hospital food.

Still, the effect of dietary manipulation on rheumatoid arthritis remains uncertain, partly because the trials that have been done are small, haven't been replicated, and have a moderate to high risk of bias, according to a review of the evidence in the *Cochrane Database of Systematic Reviews,* which typically takes a very skeptical view. That said, the authors did note that results from single trials with a moderate risk of bias indicate that fasting followed by a vegetarian diet and a Mediterranean diet "may improve pain."

Scandinavia has supplied a significant portion of the science linking diet changes to improvement in RA symptoms. Part of the reason may be cultural. People in Sweden tend to be curious about how food can affect rheumatic diseases, says Linda Hagfors, an associate professor at Umeå University in Sweden and one of the authors of the Mediterranean diet study, in an email. Swedes often experiment with vegetarian diets when they spend time at health resorts, some of which are part of the public healthcare system. But even in Scandinavian countries, studies looking at the effect of food on RA pretty much petered out just after Hagfors published her study. Why? The development of more effective drugs for rheumatoid arthritis has perhaps made getting funding for diet studies more difficult, Hagfors says.

For his part, Dr. Fischer says that because there's no way to get gold-standard evidence on diet, there's no way to be persuaded by a study of it. And how do you stop someone in a diet study from going out and getting a slice of pizza? Dr. Fischer asks. Terry Wahls, of course, had this exact problem with one of her trial participants. Science, it turns out, can sometimes be no match for gooey cheese on bread.

It doesn't help that the study of nutrition can seem a little dowdy, something like the opposite of cutting edge. This is odd considering that what we eat has everything to do with the microbiome—our community of microorganisms that lives in and on the human body— which is arguably the hottest topic in biomedical research. In 2016, the White House Office of Science and Technology Policy launched the National Microbiome Initiative to further our understanding of the microbes that live on our bodies and everywhere.

BUILDING A HEALTHY MICROBIOME

Along with infection and antibiotics, food is one of the primary ways we can alter our own population of microbes, which are found mainly in our guts. When we eat, we're feeding those guys, too.

But the key—and this is important—is to eat foods that contain fiber: vegetables, fruits, seeds, nuts, legumes, and grains that haven't been processed, that are still themselves. Offering fiber—the part of the plant that remains after our small intestine has digested what it can—to the bacteria in our large intestine was the bargain we made with them, as Dr. Fasano said. You can stay, but I hope you don't mind leftovers.

And they don't. Our bacteria thrive on fiber. Things like raspberries, pears, lentils, black beans, bran, artichokes, and green beans are all good sources according to the Mayo Clinic. Certain kinds of whole foods support certain kinds of bacteria. So eating a range of high-fiber foods is key to promoting diversity in our ranks, that crucial factor in our health.

More On What We Get Out of the Deal

We get an additional benefit from our bacteria's *digestion* of fiber. One kind of by-product of this process is short-chain fatty acids. These are essential for maintaining the integrity of the gut epithelial lining, Mayo Clinic's Veena Taneja says. Short-chain fatty acids may also prevent or ameliorate disease by helping the intestine accumulate inflammation-dampening cells, as Justin and Erica Sonnenburg write in *The Good Gut.*

The care and feeding of her gut bacteria is a possible factor in Terry Wahls's recovery, too. Though she left out whole grains and legumes, no one ate more fiber than she did. In a 2015 study in the journal *Immunity,* mice with MS-like symptoms improved after treatment with the short-chain fatty acids that bacteria produce from digesting fiber. Diet "might have therapeutic implications for auto-immune diseases such as multiple sclerosis," the authors wrote.

Beyond these pluses, scientists are starting to zero in on the roles that specific microbes may have in fighting diseases. A particular *Prevotella* species, for example, which is elevated in vegetarians, has been shown to halt or prevent RA and MS in mice. "I'm a proponent of the vegetarian diet," says Veena Taneja, who did the research. She points out that in India, where she is from, many people are vegetarians, and the severity of arthritis is less than it is in the United States.

While we work out the science of how food and bacteria affect inflammation, experimenting individually with diet makes sense, Taneja says. "That is something which doesn't hurt in any way. There are studies in mice which work in humans and there are studies which don't work. But that's the thing, we have to try."

If diet affects our microbiomes so profoundly, and we know that our microbiome affects our health profoundly, shouldn't there be more interest in studying food? "I agree!" she says. But as a scientist she also knows how hard it is to change a patient's behavior, which is why she's hoping that if that MS/RA-halting bacterium is effective in humans, it can be given to people as a pill.

Still, she would like to do a study looking at how different diets affect the mice that she's rigged to have human immune systems. "I can look at the effect of diet," Taneja says. "I want to do those studies. The only thing is, unless or until I get money I probably won't be able to do it!"

JAMIE WASN'T SPENDING ANY TIME mulling over why she felt better after only a couple of days on her new vegan diet. She was on a spree. She had never been a runner but now she started running. "I can't even describe it. All of a sudden I had strength and energy and I felt like I could be myself for the first time in a long time."

During her reprieve from arthritis she kept after her childhood goal of covering hard news. She was freelancing now as a TV traffic reporter. She would pester every boss about getting a crack at a breaking story. While she was doing a stint at News 12 New Jersey, a family had lost everything in a house fire. Jamie was sent to the charred scene to report on the tragedy.

Soon after the report aired Jamie had a meeting with her boss. She expected it to be a review of what went wrong and what went right, but mostly what went right. What he said was that he couldn't have her doing hard news on his channel. She'd reported that someone's house had burned down, and she'd smiled the entire time. "Stick to traffic," he told her.

It was crushing to the little girl with Christiane Amanpour dreams, but Jamie came to agree with the advice. It was true that she was a person who couldn't stop smiling.

She'd started her vegan diet in 2007. She had a great three years. In 2008, she and her boyfriend got engaged. On Valentine's Day. In Paris. By 2010, she had embraced her strength and was hired to be the permanent traffic anchor at New York 1, where she is today. That same year she ran the New York City half marathon.

Not long after, though, she began to feel pain in the back of her head. Around this same time, problems in her relationship emerged. After ten years together, she and her fiancé broke up.

One day, while she was jogging along the West Side Highway near her apartment in Manhattan, she had to stop. It felt as if her skull had been packed with explosives—and they were going off.

As a result of prior inflammation, the bones in her neck had become destabilized. With increased mobility comes the risk of spinal cord and nerve damage. She needed surgery to fuse two of her vertebrae so they couldn't injure her spinal cord. Jamie, being Jamie, wasn't discouraged or nervous about surgery involving her spinal cord. She zeroed in on the promise that her neck wouldn't hurt anymore. She said, "Sweet!"

After the procedure, Helen was standing over her daughter when she came to. As soon as she saw that Jamie could move her arms and legs, she started crying with relief.

Jamie was excited to get back to her life. It had been about ten months since she'd broken off her engagement. During that time she'd become a prolific dater. One day after surgery she was open again for business. The back of her head had been shaved, she was wearing a neck brace, and she had tubes coming out of her, but she picked up her phone and left a message for some guy she liked.

That was when Brian burst into her room. Brian Stelter had been on Jamie's dating roster since January—it was now July—but had had trouble climbing the rankings despite some nice dinners out together.

He'd been in touch with Jamie's friend since the surgery, asking when he could visit the hospital. Jamie told her trusted lieutenant, "Just ignore him and he won't be able to come in."

And now here he was. He was a little sweaty and a little out of breath. He was holding flowers that he'd picked up at the corner bodega.

Jamie's friend said, "I couldn't stop him."

Jamie's mom said, "I love him!"

It was the first time Brian met Helen, and he was wearing makeup. He had just come from a TV appearance. He was the television reporter for *The New York Times* and a frequent commentator on cable shows. He'd raced over to the hospital, afraid of missing visiting hours. He told Helen, "I don't normally wear makeup."

Like any respectable media couple, Jamie and Brian met on Twitter. He'd been visiting family in Maryland for Christmas. One day, like every other day, he was scanning his Twitter feed. There she was, talking about a transit shutdown.

Now, while he was in Maryland, Brian didn't exactly *need* New York transportation information, but he was drawn to it nonetheless. A huge snowstorm had just unloaded itself on the place he called home. Snow always did great things for the city, cleaning it up and quieting it down—giving it better manners. Snow invited stillness. And cross-country skiers. So as Brian tracked the storm, he was feeling like many of us do when we leave for the holidays and see people in news clips gliding down Broadway: a little left out.

Brian started following Jamie on Twitter. Soon he was tumbling through her recent tweets. And before the day was over he'd sent a message to Jamie's colleague Pat Kiernan, the NY1 anchor, whom Brian had written about in the *Times*.

He wrote, "Two innocent and unrelated questions. Does Jamie Shupak have a boyfriend? And how often is she asked out by viewers?"

Brian was feeling newly confident. He'd just lost a hundred pounds, which had changed his dating calculations. The overweight kid who'd spent his college years blogging from his dorm room about TV news felt he was cute for the first time in his adult life.

Pat Kiernan got right back to him. Yes, Jamie was single. And she was getting more attention from male viewers lately.

Brian says now that he liked her because he liked her tweets. To which she says, "Please. There's a little picture of me next to them." Brian says, "She was really cute." But there was also this: "She's also a traffic reporter in one of the biggest markets in the country." It was like a comic book geek meeting Wonder Woman.

Brian sent Jamie a message over Twitter asking her to drinks. They met at the *Times* hangout Bar Centrale on Forty-sixth Street. Drinks turned into dinner. They had a great time on that and more nights that January.

Around Valentine's Day, Brian asked Jamie to be his girlfriend.

Jamie answered: "Nope. Not a chance." She explained that she had just gotten out of a decadelong relationship. "Not locking anything down yet," she said.

One night in late September, a few months after Jamie's neck surgery, they ended up chatting on the phone for two hours. They talked about wanting one day to leave the New York media world behind and move to a farm. Jamie said she'd wear overalls every day; she already had a pair. Brian suggested she wear them the next night for the date they had planned.

She did. They had a picnic in Central Park on the grass just outside the venue where Ray LaMontagne was performing. There was something about the comfort of being with Brian. And before Jamie got home, before, even, they'd finished the weird salads-in-a-cup they'd picked up at the grocery store, she realized she was never going to be with anybody else. The glimmering New York skyline was showing off right in front of her, but she barely noticed.

They moved in together a year later and were engaged a year after that. In the year leading up to the wedding, Brian moved to CNN to become the host of *Reliable Sources.* He published a book, *Top of the Morning.* Jamie wrote her own book, a digital novel, called *Transit Girl,* and started a food blog called *TV Dinner,* which evolved into a Web video series. She appeared on the cover of *Arthritis Today,* the bold, hot-pink letters of the magazine title a perfect match to her lipstick. The cover line read: "Traffic Anchor Jamie Shupak Thrives with RA."

She *was* thriving. But she'd also been feeling arthritis pain again. This was when her ankle started to hurt, and it kept getting worse.

For her wedding she bought gold three-inch pumps to wear with her dress. She had to change out of them as soon as she walked down the aisle. She wore cowboy boots with her lacy dress for the rest of the night. Everyone thought it was a fashion choice. But if she'd actually had a choice, she would have picked the heels.

They had a Jewish ceremony, but Brian insisted they add the traditional Christian lines "in sickness and in health" to their vows. "You're marrying someone who has this battle," he says. "You gotta know that fully so that you don't hurt them in that way," he says. "I think I was very clear-eyed about it."

The difficulty with her ankle felt like a new low. The neck issue had resolved with the surgery, and she'd gotten pretty used to having fused wrists. She'd even learned to open jars by banging them just so, followed by a maneuver involving the grip of her teeth. "You figure it out if you want to live," Jamie says.

But the ankle was different. "I want to be able to walk. Forget walk! I want to be running around healthy, strong, and active," she tells me.

Unlike the problems in her other joints, this one was a lot more obvious to everyone around her. "When you limp, everyone looks at you," she says. "It's not even in a mean way, but everyone's eyes go directly to the limp. You're different." It was the constant reminder that was hard.

Having trouble walking was also freighted with symbolism. When she and Brian went away for a weekend to Boston, Brian suggested they catch the airport's courtesy golf cart to get to their gate. She laid into him. That was for handicapped people, and she wasn't handicapped. She could walk. He pointed out that it hurt when she walked. Why not use something to make her life easier? "Yeah, but I can walk so I'm going to keep walking until my foot's like, 'You can't walk anymore,'" she said. "It's almost like once you get on you're never going to get off," she tells me.

At the same time she realized she needed to fix her ankle, she felt that she had come to the end of what her doctor could do for her. She still trusted Dr. Fischer, but she found his ideas for treatment limited to trying other drug therapies. Having cycled through so many that hadn't worked, she was no longer optimistic about their potential. Plus she'd started to worry about the long-term effects the drugs, especially the newest ones that lacked a track record, would have on her body. And she still wasn't content with treating just the symptoms.

It was almost like outgrowing a romantic relationship that had started when she was too young. She'd changed. There was a bigger world out there.

She realized that if she wanted to try anything out-of-the-box, experimental, or odd, regular physicians weren't going to participate. It all fell into the alternative medicine category, but alternative to what? Nothing else had worked for her.

She started acting like a primary care doctor, overseeing her own care. Dr. Fischer was just one of several people she was now listening to, even though his information had the most evidence behind it. "You get advice from three different people and it's all very different advice. Here we are sitting on a couch deciding what medicines I should take or try!"

It was the Internet, of course, that made her role possible, granting her access to other sources of information. Since she'd been diagnosed, the culture had changed, too. Jamie, like everyone else, had become more demanding about getting facts immediately. It helped that Jamie and Brian were journalists, trained to dig and practiced at sizing up whatever was found. "Brian is a Google ninja!" Jamie says.

The problem is that when you're on the frontier, there is, by definition, nothing proven that you're going to find. Brian found himself giving anecdotal evidence and educated guesses more weight than he would have had he been reporting on it. There were different rules when it was family and you were desperate, as I discovered myself.

He realized that if he was going to question Eastern medicine or other unproven therapies, he also had to take a hard look at drugs. "One of the biggest *aha* moments for me through the past few years has been when she was in a couple of these arthritis magazines. I probably shouldn't say this, but it really seems like these magazines prioritize and emphasize drugs as opposed to other possibilities. That's not a coincidence," he says, referring to the money those magazines and the foundations that publish them receive from pharmaceutical companies. Ads from drugmakers are an important source of revenue for medical journals, too, according to the Pew Charitable Trusts. "That makes me think about the limits of what we would consider the mainstream, to understand the implications there, to understand the driving forces."

Meanwhile Jamie was busy making her own interpretations. She felt that if an intervention helped one person, maybe it could help another. She knew this was a rickety proposition, but still.

I asked Derek Lowe, a medical chemist who's worked in drug discovery for three decades and writes the *In the Pipeline* blog on the topic, if there is any value to a single success story from where he sat. "One time is no time," Lowe told me, quoting a German expression. "Every decent scientist knows that." Fair enough. But when it comes to buying hope, as I discovered myself, one positive outcome goes pretty far. "That's the thing with hope. You only need one," Terry Wahls's son, Zach, told me.

Like other people in this book, Jamie would not accept that she couldn't beat her disease—never considered it. There had to be an answer out there for her problem, even if she had to be the one to figure it out.

SEAMUS MULLEN

There was one name that kept turning up in Jamie's online searches for stories about overcoming rheumatoid arthritis: Seamus Mullen, a chef whose reimagining of Spanish cuisine made him a star on the New York City food scene and a regular on the Food Network.

For years he'd felt run-down and achy. His hands and one of his shoulders would hurt, but he was also working ninety hours a week in the kitchen. Then one morning, Seamus awoke to excruciating pain in his hip. A neighbor heard him screaming and found him on the floor. He was admitted to the hospital and the screaming lasted for several more days. He was diagnosed with rheumatoid arthritis.

It was his grandmother who first suggested he think about what he was eating. "She said, 'Listen, you're a chef. You should really think about how food impacts you. I bet that there's a correlation,'" Seamus tells me. "Her perspective was very much the old school, you are what you eat."

So Seamus did his own research and discovered that some of the central components of the Spanish food he loved—olive oil and anchovies, for example—were thought to be anti-inflammatory. He began talking about eating his way to health. He wrote a cookbook called *Seamus Mullen's Hero Food*, championing the same idea. And he did feel better after cutting out processed foods and alcohol and zeroing in on whole foods and a lot of healthy fats—who wouldn't? But the truth was, he told me later, he was still struggling. He knew that eating well was fundamental to being healthy, but it wasn't enough.

He told himself he would do whatever it took to be healthy. "Whatever the work is, I will do it." But there was one problem with that. He realized, *I really don't know what that work is.*

He met someone who had some suggestions, not about controlling symptoms but about treating whatever was causing his autoimmune disorder.

FUNCTIONAL MEDICINE

A mutual friend had introduced Seamus to Dr. Frank Lipman, who practices functional medicine, an emerging subspecialty situated in the broader category of integrative medicine. In 2014, the Cleveland Clinic opened the Center for Functional Medicine, the first major medical institution to do so.

Functional medicine doctors describe themselves as looking for the cause of illness, which kind of sounds like a joke. Isn't that what all physicians are supposed to do?

I put that question to Dr. Susan S. Blum, a functional medicine practitioner and an assistant clinical professor in the department of preventive medicine at the Icahn School of Medicine at Mount Sinai in New York. She says all doctors are trained to *treat* patients, but there are differences in their understanding of what that means.

"Traditional training is focused on trying to treat the symptoms related to the disease, so that people feel better. For a rheumatologist, the *cause* of the joint pain is inflammation, and the *cause* of the inflammation is the overactive/dysfunctional immune system. Suppress the immune system, and—voilà!—they can treat the patient's symptoms." So they are treating the inflammation, the cause of the pain.

But functional medicine doctors like Dr. Blum argue that that's secondary. She looks for the primary cause: Why is the immune system not working right to begin with? "We are detectives and we keep looking."

Seamus says that Dr. Lipman was different from any doctor he had ever met because Dr. Lipman wanted to listen. "I read that seventeen seconds is the average amount of time that a doctor waits before he stops listening to you," Seamus says. Dr. Lipman told him, "I want to know what's going on with you." According to a 2005 study, 37 percent of doctors observed failed to ask what was wrong in the first five minutes. These doctors were far less likely to identify the problem, the authors wrote in the *Journal of General Internal Medicine.*

But doctors—particularly primary care doctors—have also become squeezed for time with patients, and they don't like it any more than you do. One major reason for compressed appointments is the considerable administrative burden that comes with practicing medicine today, especially for those who accept insurance, which Dr. Lipman does not. In 2014, doctors reported spending 20 percent of their time on paperwork alone, according to a survey by the Physicians Foundation.

After Seamus talked for nearly an hour, Dr. Lipman asked him to go home and write down his full medical history going back to childhood. He wanted to know everything, and he wanted supporting documentation where possible.

Dr. Lipman believed that Seamus's arthritis started with a compromised bacteria population. Although our friend Dr. Fasano used more cautious language when speculating about what he thought led to Shepherd's arthritis—"it's possible," "could be linked," "might have started"—the scenario Dr. Fasano described was similar.

Dr. Lipman told Seamus that he suspected his gut flora started getting screwed up in high school when he had a salmonella infection and antibiotics were used to treat it. Over time, he said to Seamus, you started eating a traditional American simple carbohydrate–based, sugary diet. But because you were young and healthy, says Seamus, paraphrasing Dr. Lipman, you were able to deal with it. Then you got really sick in Mexico and I suspect you probably got parasites. You've got a bacterial imbalance going on in your gut. Probably being driven largely by parasites, being reinforced by not such a healthy diet. You developed excessive gut permeability and bacteria's going into your bloodstream.

He sent Seamus to get checked for parasites, and, sure enough, he tested positive. Dr. Lipman started Seamus on a course of heavy-duty Western meds, including antiparasitics, at the same time that he had Seamus radically change his diet. Seamus was already off alcohol. Dr. Lipman suggested he also cut sugar, dairy, and grains—not just those that contained gluten. Dr. Lipman tells me that he often sees other grains causing problems in autoimmune diseases, and there are plenty of other sources of fiber. Seamus himself added legumes to the banned-foods list.

"It literally was six months to the day," says Seamus. "I woke up one morning and my hands weren't stiff and swollen."

Again, we don't know why Seamus got better, but there's plenty to speculate about. Like Shepherd and Terry Wahls, Seamus cut out possible leaky gut instigators, such as dairy and gluten, and added in plenty of rich-in-fiber whole foods—bacteria comfort food.

Rheumatologists say we haven't yet figured out the cause of— or the cure for—autoimmune arthritis. "There's evidence suggesting that it starts in the gut," says Jamie's rheumatologist, Dr. Fischer. "There's clearly a relationship, but we haven't really defined it. I think it's still unknown."

Functional medicine doctors like Dr. Lipman are obviously less conservative. He evidently didn't feel compelled to wait for better evidence. Plenty of people, according to Dr. Lipman, call him a quack.

*　　*　　*

JAMIE KEPT READING ABOUT SEAMUS. In more recent stories, Seamus talked about being off medication and about the doctor who'd helped him get there. Jamie recognized Dr. Lipman's name. He was the guy Gwyneth Paltrow was always talking about. (Jamie was a consumer of food, health, and fitness blogs, a genre that she describes as being centered on what various celebrities were putting in their smoothies.) Dr. Lipman was also a contributor to the actress's loved/hated lifestyle website Goop.

Here was her next source! Jamie called Dr. Lipman's office. Given that an Oscar winner was a patient, Jamie suspected it could be difficult to get an appointment. So when the receptionist asked Jamie if anyone had referred her, she said, having never met him, "Seamus Mullen?" The receptionist said, "Great. How about Tuesday?"

Dr. Lipman's plan for Jamie, as it had been with Seamus, was to identify what might be wreaking havoc in her gut—creating imbalance among the bacteria—and then use medication and a grain-free, dairy-free, sugar-free, alcohol-free diet to restore the situation down there. The idea was to promote a variety of good bacteria by feeding it a variety of good fiber.

Shortly after her appointment with Dr. Lipman, she called one of Seamus's restaurants and got his email address. He responded right away. They met and talked for hours. "I wrote down every single thing he's ever put in his body."

Again she went whole hog, combining the advice she got from Dr. Lipman and from Seamus about what to eat and which supplements to take (probiotics, fish oil, various herbs). She'd already cut alcohol, as a vegan she avoided dairy, and she'd never eaten a lot of sugar. So her new, restricted diet didn't feel so restricted, actually. She became buddies with free-range, organic chicken, eggs, and bacon. For breakfast she made green shakes for herself and Brian—kale or spinach, apple or pineapple, almond milk, almond butter, fibrous chia and hemp seeds, cinnamon, and assorted supplements. She ate big salads topped with every kind of vegetable, nut, seed, and fruit. She even found a recipe for grain-free chocolate chip cookies.

Again she felt better. She had more energy, and the pain in all of her joints except for her foot faded away. She'd recently started feeling arthritis in one of her shoulders, but that went away, too. When a stool test showed she had the same parasite her new friend Seamus had had—the thing Dr. Lipman attributed his RA to—she was thrilled. "Yeah!" she said, in what was likely the first time old *Entamoeba histolytica* has been greeted so warmly. "He's better. I'm going to get better. This is amazing!"

Dr. Lipman gave Jamie strong antibiotics, but when they didn't seem to affect her arthritis, he told her that the drugs hadn't been able to wipe out the parasite. Next up was the antiparasitic Seamus had also been on—for months. They made Jamie ragingly nauseous for a couple of days. "I can do it. I can do it. I can do it," she told herself. Until she woke up to a level of world-spinning queasiness she'd never known. She had to pull the plug.

She and Brian met again with Dr. Lipman. Since changing her diet she definitely felt better overall. It was plain to her that drinking alcohol and eating certain foods, namely dairy, made her joints feel worse. Regardless of how disciplined she was with food, though, her ankle was still a wreck.

That's when Dr. Lipman mentioned a fecal transplant. It was basically all he had left.

Fecal Microbiota Transplantation and Autoimmune Disease

Dr. Lipman told them that the procedure had been uncommonly successful in people with *C. diff* infections, that kind of bacteria that causes severe diarrhea. When stool from healthy donors is transferred to the intestines of these patients, usually via colonoscopy, balance is almost always restored to their guts. The replenished population of bacteria seems to be able to rein in the deadly ones.

Given that Dr. Lipman believed a compromised bacterial population was at play with Jamie's rheumatoid arthritis, he felt that a fecal transplant could help her, too. This was pure theory. To his knowledge, no one had tried a fecal transplant for RA. As of this writing the FDA allows the procedure, formally referred to as fecal microbiota transplantation, or FMT, for recurrent *C. diff* infections only.

There is some evidence in mice that suggests that restoring a healthy gut bacteria population could be therapeutic for autoimmune conditions. Mice without a microbiota have a disrupted immune system, the Stanford microbiologist Erica Sonnenburg writes me in an email. "Adding back a microbiota can restore normal immune system function (assuming the timing is early enough in development)." Because there are no bacteria-free humans, though, we can't try to replicate the results in people. "But," Sonnenburg says, "there is growing evidence that fecal transplants, which are a way of restoring the microbiota, have promise in treating diseases such as obesity, diabetes, and inflammatory bowel disease, which have in common a disrupted immune response."

Scientists at the major research universities are eager to do more trials, but before they can proceed, they need permission from the FDA as well as approval from their own institutions and all of the individual departments involved. While science revs its engine, bureaucracy can sit on the brake pedal.

Dr. Alexander Khoruts, the gastroenterologist and associate professor of medicine at the University of Minnesota, was the first to get permission from the FDA to study FMT in *C. diff* patients. His application papers weighed twenty-two pounds. For a new study looking at FMT in prediabetic patients, the approval process took a full year and a half. Even the arduous task of procuring funding for such a trial was faster. With NIH financing for clinical trials so scarce, Dr. Khoruts went to the state of Minnesota, which had set aside funding for the environment. He argued rather ingeniously that our microbiomes were ecosystems facing extinction.

While the research is held up, regular people are forging ahead on their own even though they don't know if it will work or what the risks are. The Internet is loaded with stories of people, typically with GI (gastrointestinal) tract issues, trying fecal transplants at home, enema-style. "There are a lot of desperate people because standard medicine has not provided them with adequate treatment," says Dr. Khoruts. "That this is happening tells you that something is wrong. It should be easier than that to get medical guidance. If these trials are not happening because of barriers that are put up, that's a problem."

Dr. Lipman told Jamie that if she could find someone that would give her a fecal transplant, even though they're not approved for RA patients, he thought it could help her. She and Brian left the appointment half-excited about the prospect and half-stunned that they'd already tapped out the doctor. *He's out? That was it? We ran through all of his ideas?* Jamie thought as they walked out of the office. *Wait! I'm not better yet!*

It was a very real moment, she says. "Wait. We came to you because you were the guy. And now that's it? It's really fucking scary and sad when you're done with someone because then it's like, what now?"

But they weren't done, not yet. Jamie thought Brian's reaction to the fecal transplant idea was going to be "FUCK NO!" But instead, his eyes seemed to light up a little, she says. Jamie pounced. "Oh my God! I'm GETTING it! I am flying to fucking Australia if that's where they'll replace my poop and doing it."

Now that a fecal transplant was on the table, sensei Brian did a lot of googling. There was nothing out there about RA patients. It really looked like Jamie would be the first, but he found himself still open to it. The press coverage of fecal transplants in general was reassuring. Also, there seemed to be a lack of downside, he says. It wasn't dangerous, as far as anyone knew. But that's different from *knowing* that it wasn't risky, which wasn't the case, given the lack of data.

Fixing her arthritis had taken on new urgency because she and Brian were eager to have a baby. As many of us in this book have discovered, children were a great motivator, perhaps the greatest. "I wanna be a healthy, strong mom," she wrote to me in one email. "Who can walk!"

Then Jamie got an email from Dr. Lipman. "Poop guy. Heard he's doing RA." He gave her the name and number of a gastroenterologist who lived in another state.

Now that the fecal transfer was a real possibility, Jamie had to consider if she was really up for self-experimentation. And she was. "I don't care if I have this and I'm limping every day for the rest of my life," she says. "I just want to know that I did everything that was humanly possible. If I don't keep trying, what am I doing with my life?" And, who knows, Jamie wondered, maybe in that effort someone would benefit from what she did. Maybe she could supply an anecdote that could get a researcher's attention.

Young and otherwise healthy, she thought she was a good candidate. Plus Dr. Lipman wasn't worried. And she'd tried something—the chemotherapy infusion—that had a risk of death. What could be worse than that?

Jamie describes Dr. Lipman as "an incredible human." She tells me, "Be prepared to be a believer in everything that comes outta his mouth." This is striking because it shows how trust in a doctor is no longer a given. It has to do with faith.

She forwards me Dr. Lipman's response to her request that he talk to me: "Of course, Hon. I will do anything for you . . . you are such a gem. Keep me posted on the poop."

In a 2008 study in the *BMJ*, patients who got more attention from doctors fared better. A sample of people with irritable bowel syndrome were divided into three groups. The first received no treatment, but 28 percent of the patients still improved after three weeks. The second group received fake acupuncture and spoke to the doctor for only five minutes; 44 percent of them felt better. The last set of patients got the sham treatment along with forty-five minutes of warm, empathetic conversation with the doctor: "I can understand how difficult IBS must be for you." These doctors also projected confidence and expertise. A remarkable 62 percent of the patients who got this kind of care—with no treatment—reported improved symptoms. Of these three dimensions of the placebo effect—spontaneous recovery, belief in a sham treatment, and that faith coupled with kind doctoring—the researchers concluded that "the patient-practitioner relationship is the most robust component." This seems kind of amazing, too—the factors contributing to the placebo effect could be added to each other like upping the dose of a drug, the researchers wrote.

When I meet Dr. Lipman, he leads me down a warmly lit hallway, curved like an enormous parenthesis, to his office. "From a Western perspective, rheumatoid arthritis and all autoimmune diseases, they don't really treat the cause," he says. "They just treat the symptoms, and they give toxic drugs to do that. Where I come from, from a functional medicine perspective, rheumatoid arthritis and autoimmune diseases in general, you're looking for the cause. The cause is often coming from the gut. I'm not saying I know. I've just seen enough people clinically get better when I've done what I've done to know, to know—not to believe—to know that the way we do this in Western medicine is really not only—maybe it helps some people—but it harms a lot of people. I really think it behooves us as medical practitioners to actually look for the cause and actually try to treat people without harming them."

Conventional rheumatologists argue that not treating inflammatory arthritis right away with medications that are proven to work puts the patient at risk. "We don't want to see a joint get irreversibly injured," says Jamie's rheumatologist, Dr. Fischer.

One of the more conspicuous things about the functional medicine specialist Dr. Lipman is the number of times he uses words like "guesswork" and "crapshoot" and "chance," which, because he is from South Africa, he pronounces *chonce.* He has an unusual comfort with not knowing that a given treatment will work, though no one knows definitely that a medication is going to affect an individual, either. "All I can say for sure," he says, "is that there's usually a gut component to these autoimmune problems like rheumatoid arthritis. How you actually treat it is very difficult because everyone's different, and you're guessing. Sometimes you guess right. Sometimes it takes months. We've had major success stories."

He says he encouraged Jamie to try a fecal transplant because it made so much sense to him, despite the lack of science in the case of RA patients. "Why not try? If you're going to try biologics, why don't you try a fecal transplant first?" he says. "Hospital medicine is fantastic. It saves lives. Chronic disease? Western medicine is not particularly helpful. It's a Band-Aid. And the Band-Aid often causes problems."

"The idea of fecal transplants," he says, "is very intriguing and should be explored, but there's no big money. No drug company is going to make money on it, so who's going to put money behind it? We have a money-driven system, so it's not about the good of the patient. It's about the good of the pharmaceutical industry. It's screwed up! I think fecal transplants are the future of medicine. It's crazy that you can't"—*con't*—"do it. They legalize these toxic drugs and not something like a fecal transplant, which is not expensive."

Holly Campbell, a spokesperson for PhRMA, the pharmaceutical industry trade association, responds, saying, "Innovative treatments are transforming care for patients fighting debilitating diseases like cancer, hepatitis C, high cholesterol, and more."

Antiarthritic drugs are certainly great for business. In 2013, they brought in more than $15 billion, according to QuintilesIMS, a healthcare information, services, and technology solutions company.

Dr. Lipman himself is not a bystander to the marketplace. He sells his own products, including the $239 Be Well by Dr. Frank Lipman cleanse, fourteen days' worth of prepackaged shakes and supplements. He's become something of a celebrity guru. Just beneath the "add to cart" button on his website, the actress Maggie Gyllenhaal is quoted saying, "I eat what he tells me to eat and drink what he tells me to drink."

I ask Dr. Fischer, Jamie's rheumatologist, if he thought the research emphasis on pharmaceuticals was in the right place. Are we investing in the most promising therapies? "I think that we've made such great strides," he says. "How could I not say that?" He tells me that when he was a fellow, he used to regularly see patients in wheelchairs. These days that's very rare.

For people like Jamie, who haven't had much luck with medication, the pharmaceutical industry is working on new chances. There are currently forty medicines in development for RA alone, according to Holly Campbell, the PhRMA spokesperson.

✿   ✿   ✿

WHEN JAMIE TRIED TO EXTRACT a blessing from her rheumatologist for the fecal transplant, he was not forthcoming. Because there was no data, Dr. Fischer told her it was impossible to know the risks. She asked him if he thought it could kill her. He allowed that he didn't think so. At worst, she would probably get stomach upset. Okay, then.

Jamie and Brian arranged for a consultation with the out-of-state gastroenterologist. He told them he'd never tried a transplant on a patient with RA but that he was very interested to see how it would work. It actually *was* pretty pricey. For $2,000, she could have it done in his offices via enema. And then, not without enthusiasm, he told her he knew exactly who they were going to use as her donor. Jamie thought: "You don't even know me!" The donor was in her twenties and trying to get pregnant, so she was being diligent about her health. She'd been a successful donor for them thus far for *C. diff* and other patients. "I don't even want to know how much poop this girl has donated or what she's getting in return," says Jamie.

The gastroenterologist explained that a fecal transplant via colonoscopy, which is how it's usually performed, was approved only for patients with *C. diff*, which is why he was offering an enema. He told her that because of the regulations, she was supposed to give it to herself and that he would be there to guide her through the procedure. At least, officially. "He was sort of like, 'Wink. Wink. We do it for you behind closed doors. But we tell people that we're just showing you how to do it.'" Meanwhile Jamie was thinking, "If I'm paying two thousand dollars, you're sticking it in me! I'm not putting it . . . I don't even . . . NO. No."

The gastroenterologist does not dispute Jamie's account. In fact, he asked not to be identified so that his clinic would not get shut down. "We try to stay within the guidelines," he tells me. "But we bend the rules."

He says that his clinic has branched out into doing fecal transplants for unapproved diseases and conditions because people have tapped out other options and are desperate. "It's very early to make a big statement about this, but we've seen that there has been benefit in certain autoimmune disorders. And we feel in disorders that are triggered by antibiotic use and disruption of the microbiome, such as ulcerative colitis and Crohn's disease, correcting that problem"—restoring bacteria via FMT—"has been beneficial. If you want to extrapolate to other autoimmune diseases—RA, psoriasis, lupus—there is potential benefit there. Clearly there need to be more studies done. But given the safety and potential benefit, it was worth trying."

I ask if we really know at this point that it's safe. "We know that this has been done since 1958," he says. "If you scour the literature, you'd be hard-pressed to find any major complications other than maybe some bloating, burping, or a transient low-grade fever." To mitigate potential problems down the road, the clinic does rigorous screening. You can't be a donor if your family has any history of cancer, autoimmune disease, or obesity, among other diseases. No wonder the clinic has only three people contributing.

As Jamie contemplated getting the world's most expensive enema, she heard from Dr. Lipman again: "I heard he's doing the pills. Call him." Sure enough, the gastroenterologist would be happy to send her, instead, capsules filled with fecal matter. They were half the price of the enema, but there was also a greater risk that the capsules' contents wouldn't make it to their destination in the gut; stomach acid could easily kill bacteria if it breached the capsule. The gastroenterologist explains to me that there are three layers of capsules to each pill. Plus, he says, the fact that almost 90 percent of his *C. diff* patients who've taken the pills have recovered is evidence that the bacteria within the capsules are getting to where they need to go. Those who receive the transplant via colonoscopy have a higher cure rate—99 percent.

The smaller commitment of the pills appealed to Jamie. The doctor gave Jamie the initials of that young donor he'd mentioned before. He told Jamie to be sure to tell his assistant that's who they were going to use. Jamie kept thinking about her. "I kept thinking if she makes it so I can walk again, I am meeting this woman, girl, whatever."

While Jamie was definitely excited about this new chance at recovery, she still had her down days. She worried about how she was going to take

care of a baby if she continued to have limited dexterity and trouble walking. She would watch moms in her neighborhood. "I look at the strollers
and the car seats, your hands doing all that stuff all the time."

She worries about the effect that her arthritis has on Brian. She'll
tell him, "It's not because I think that you don't love me or whatever.
I just think that you didn't sign up for this." Brian tells her, "Everyone
has a thing. You're worried about the buckles on car seats and things?
We will fucking invent a car seat that you don't need those for! We'll
figure it out."

He tells me, "She will claim that her hands are ugly. I genuinely on
a stack of Bibles believe her hands are one of her five best features.
Maybe I have a hand fetish, I don't know! I think I believed it before
I noticed that sometimes her hands swell up, her fingers swell up.
She'll never believe this stuff, but it's so deeply rooted in me."

I MEET JAMIE FOR THE first time the day after her pills arrive. She'd
agreed to let me be there for their debut.

She pulls the brown paper bag out of the freezer and opens it up.
There's a letter inside. "Keep capsules frozen at all times. Take two
frozen capsules a day with a glass of water at mealtime." The instructions are printed out on a piece of regular white paper with no letter-
head. It's not signed. "That's it?" Jamie says. "I guess what else are you
going to say?" Later, she'll refer to it as a ransom note.

She unscrews the lid and instinctively takes a whiff. This makes
me laugh. She reports that there's no odor, which I can confirm. We
both examine the capsules containing what appears to be frozen light
brown liquid.

Then she says, "Are we going to do it?" I tell her that "we" are not
going to do anything. I suggest she eat some of the almonds that are
in a bag on her kitchen counter because the instructions mentioned
taking the pills with food. "Poop and nuts!" she says. "It's dinner-
time!"

Once she decided to take the pills, she wasn't worried about what they would do to her. What she was worried about was that if something went wrong, she was going to have to go to the hospital and explain, "I'm eating somebody's poop."

For the first couple of days that she was taking the pills she didn't poop herself. Ironic. When she finally did, she immediately called Brian with the report. "He says he's interested," she says.

Brian tells me, "We are in the post-TMI age," as in, too much information. He goes on. "But isn't that the joy of marriage, too? You finally have someone you can say ev-er-y-thing to?"

While she was still taking the pills, she saw an orthopedist about her ankle. She says he took a look at her and said he didn't know how she was still walking. The ankle consists of two joints: the subtalar, which allows for lateral movement, and what's called the true ankle joint, which is for up-and-down motion. Jamie's subtalar joint was bone on bone. There was no cartilage left between them. No amount of good bacteria, she knew, was going to bring that back.

The only option, once again, was surgery to fuse the two bones. As with the vertebrae in her neck, joining the two pieces would take away the pain. Her side-to-side movement would be limited, but she'd be able to walk again normally.

This was good and bad news. Good that there was an answer. Bad because there was a chance that she was pregnant. And if that was the case, she wouldn't be able to have the surgery. Meanwhile her joint was getting worse every day. "What are we going to do?" she asked Brian.

A test showed she wasn't pregnant, and she scheduled the surgery.

Jamie finished out the course of fecal pills just before she went into the hospital. While she was home for a month recovering, she was also tapering down her steroids. She'd been taking more for her ankle, but now that was no longer necessary. She was on other pain meds for the surgery so it was a good time, Dr. Fischer agreed, to try to come off some of the RA drugs. She said to him, "Look at you, trying to get me off drugs!"

Dr. Fischer had actually been keen to get her off the prednisone, specifically, for a while. There is a multitude of adverse effects from taking the drug long-term, he tells me: potential bone loss, increased risk of infection, elevation of blood sugar, and cataract formation.

Several months after the surgery, Jamie was walking without pain. The procedure was successful. The arthritis in her other joints seemed to have stabilized, too: She was able to get her dose of prednisone lower than what it had been during the almost ten years before her ankle started hurting.

It's impossible to sort out why. "We're never sure what causes flares and what settles them down," says her rheumatologist, Dr. Fischer.

As for the fecal pills, it's hard to know if they even got a real chance to make a difference. When Jamie had her subtalar joint fused—right after she finished her last capsule—she was given antibiotics. So while the bacteria-fighting drugs held down Jamie's risk of infection from the surgery, they probably also limited the potential benefit from the young woman with the $1,000 sample. After all of that.

I ask Dr. Lipman what he thinks the effect of the antibiotics was on the transplanted bacteria. It's possible it was all wiped out, he writes me in an email, "although [I] would hope to think not."

FEWER THAN TWO YEARS LATER, Jamie was back in the operating room. Inflammation had worn away the cartilage in her true ankle joint, next to where she'd had the earlier fusion in her right foot. This time, she had the entire joint replaced.

And so her confounding disease remains true to itself, its moods and whims inscrutable. But Jamie is just as unchanged. Her brightness—that RA foil—is not at all dimmed.

She tells me that she would consider trying fecal pills again but doesn't feel she needs to yet. "Right now, my body feels great, especially since fixing my one problematic joint. I'm walking like a total boss," she says. "No pain, no limp, no nothing. You would have no idea I ever had any problems or surgeries."

She's finally able to focus on getting pregnant. She wants a basketball team—five boys. Brian has a wish, too. He hopes that if his future children ever have problems, they'll be fighters like their mom. Not long ago he tweeted out a message about Jamie. It was their anniversary. He wrote: "One year ago today. She said 'I do.' I said 'I really do.'"

9

The Science of the Mind and Body

"Things Shift Toward Wellness"

IF ANYONE WAS GOING TO FEEL A PLACEBO EFFECT, THE HEALING that happens when you believe a treatment will make you better, it was Jamie.

Even though we often think of placebos as the sugar pills people are given in medical experiments, they don't have to involve a false therapy. The study in the chapter about Jamie, showing the powerful influence a doctor's confidence and kindness can have on recovery, is a great example of the other factors that can prompt a placebo effect. In fact, the placebo effect is likely to happen "just about any time you seek healing in a setting that creates an expectation of improvement," according to a 2014 Mayo Clinic report.

And now consider Jamie. She's like Pigpen from Peanuts, only instead of a dust cloud, she constantly radiates optimism. During her battle with RA, every treatment was going to work, she just knew it, and it did, usually, until it didn't. Then she was always on to the next, her hope unscathed. Amanda Hanson, too—she *expected* Hayden to heal, which no doubt rubbed off on her son. Terry Wahls was more conservative about the possibility of recovery at first, but then she became positively bullish.

Faith like that can release endorphins, those potent pain-fighting chemicals homemade by our bodies. If you've been given morphine before and then take a phony version you think is real, you'll likely feel a similar effect, according to a 1999 study in *The Journal of Neuroscience*. The relief is not in your head; you're accessing your own pharmacy. In a similar way, athletes who doped with fake morphine, after having taken the actual drug at a previous time, also got a boost, researchers reported in 2007 in the same journal. The subjects lasted longer in a pain tolerance competition, which was a stand-in for endurance sports.

This kind of expectation-as-drug following exposure to the real thing has been repeated in studies of an immune suppressant, a dopamine drug for Parkinson's, and an anti-anxiety medication.

In fact, drugs often turn out to derive a major portion of their benefit, if not all of their benefit, from positive expectations rather than the therapy itself, according to the Mayo Clinic. Surgeries, too.

Parkinson's disease is caused by the breakdown of neurons deep in the brain. Surgically implanting neurons from embryos into patients' brains has been shown to improve symptoms in a few studies. But none of these tested the surgery against placebo: believing you're getting the treatment. In a 2004 *Archives of General Psychiatry* study, Parkinson's patients underwent brain surgery but only half got the transplant. Those who believed they had gotten the new neurons— whether they had or not—did better than those who didn't believe. Doctors saw improvement in motor functioning, tremors, and walking ability, among other measures.

How a placebo works exactly is a mystery. Part of the reason is that trying to understand the connection between the mind and body has not traditionally been a major focus of biomedical research. "It's a word that we use to dismiss a lot of what happens, to factor out the role of the mind, and then we move on to the other stuff," says the Harvard psychiatrist Dr. Jeffrey Rediger. "But the mind is a huge factor in why people get better and why people respond in medical studies. We're leaving this big, gaping question that's unexamined," he says. "It's amazing, isn't it?"

Dr. Rediger's research interest is spontaneous remission—when people get better for reasons we don't understand. Dr. Rediger believes there's a strong mind component to it. As with the placebo effect, we know spontaneous remission happens, we just don't know why. "What's fascinating to me," he says, "is that there's nothing spontaneous about spontaneous remission," meaning there's probably a lot that happens in order to bring about the phenomenon. "It's just that we never asked," Dr. Rediger says—we haven't studied it enough to know what that process is.

Now, Dr. Rediger is asking. He is seeking funding for a study of people who've recovered from serious illnesses in the absence of treatment. He's talked to over one hundred people who have medical evidence of having had an incurable disease—only the hardcore cases. One woman was diagnosed by biopsy with the most fatal form of pancreatic cancer and told she was going to die. He says that records confirm that his subjects' diagnoses were correct—and that they recovered.

He's gone back to these ex-patients to try to understand what happened. Since 2003, he's conducted interviews, and though he's not finished analyzing the data, he has found that his subjects have a lot in common in terms of attitude. "I believe from talking to lots of people, and we'll see if the research bears this out, but what seems to be the case is that when people are able to have an experience of themselves—not just a cognitive thought—but an experience that they really matter more than they realized, that maybe they're not fundamentally defective individuals, but there's something there that's good and worthy, simply without qualification, or that they're less alone than they thought, there's something that can shift that can be extremely powerful," he says.

And a lot of times, the people in Dr. Rediger's proposed study have made significant dietary and lifestyle changes. "I think we're also biological beings, so I do think that food is medicine and when people begin to respect themselves enough to give something more natural to their bodies—whether the change happens at a level of biology and lifestyle, by changing what one eats, or happens at a mental level, or however one understands it—those shifts at one level often go into the other level," he says. "And things shift, it seems, towards wellness."

So it could be that eating well is significant not only for how the food nourishes the body and its bacteria, but for what it represents in terms of a person's self-respect. The act of taking care of ourselves may be healing because it signifies that we matter. "Maybe I should give up those processed foods or maybe I've got some chemicals in my life that have not been helping me or whatever it is," Dr. Rediger says. The people he wants to study who recovered, he says, at some level seemed to see themselves much more compassionately, less judgmentally than they used to. If they'd always thought they were never good enough, they realized that they had a misunderstanding.

"I deeply believe in science," he says. "But I think that science only looks at external remedies like medicines and procedures. I think it takes often a very different approach than that for a person to get genuinely healthy because I think that medicines and procedures often treat symptoms, not causes. So that's one limitation."

Dr. Rediger, who is also the chief of behavioral medicine at Good Samaritan Medical Center, says that what he's learned about spontaneous remission already is changing the way he thinks about everything as a person and a physician. "What I'm becoming convinced of is that there are aspects of mind and quote-unquote heart that are involved in many of our illnesses. And because we have such a chasm between mind and body, the way we are taught to think about medicine, we don't even know how to scientifically study aspects of mind," he says.

And then he says something even more striking. "I am the chief of psychiatry at a medical hospital and a medical director at a psychiatric hospital. I can tell you I absolutely believe that mind is driving much of the chronic illness that is eighty-five percent of the disease burden in this country," he says. "I'm not kidding you. We're talking trillions of dollars. We're talking about enormous suffering. Just the five major chronic diseases of diabetes, arthritis, lung disease, the lifestyle aspects of cancer, and heart disease—these have a huge mind component."

It's not the kind of talk you expect to hear from a medical director of a hospital affiliated with one of our most esteemed—and conservative—institutions. In fact, Dr. Rediger wasn't always this forthcoming about his understanding of a mind-body connection. "I think medicine doesn't tolerate change easily," he says. "I was nervous about it for a couple of years, nervous about being out of the closet with this way of thinking. I didn't have the confidence to be bold about it," he says.

He's faced some pushback at Harvard about his views, but he understands it. "Resistance probably occurs much or all of the time for new ideas, especially those that raise questions about new possibilities and new paradigms. In some ways, one should probably be grateful for resistance. It tests one's mettle, one's sincerity."

And he has great respect for Harvard's role, the value of its imprimatur. "Harvard is a complicated institution and while aspects within it may not always be at the forefront of change, it is probably one of the most powerful legitimizing influences in the world," he says. "Initial resistance is important, from that perspective."

Despite any professional pressure not to talk about the role of the mind in recovery, Dr. Rediger is committed to pursuing it. "I'm very good at my day job so that gives me some freedom. I've slowly become convinced that I have a responsibility to take a stand, to say this. I can't stay silent anymore," he says. "I have to do this. I can't not do this."

Like other rebellious thinkers in this book, Dr. Rediger grew up an outsider, perhaps the ultimate outsider—his family was Amish. "I was raised in the culture but not of the culture," he says. He went to public school, but at home there was no TV, no radio. His home life was extremely conservative, against science because science was evolution and that was the devil, he says. Knowledge outside of the Bible was suspect. But even as a boy his own instincts clashed with what he was being told was right and true. "Religion wasn't working for me," he says. "So I ended up being a skeptic of both science and religion." His quest to figure it out led him first to seminary at Princeton, and then to medical school because, as he says, "I became convinced that science was wonderful."

It's also conservative in its own way. Dr. Rediger understands that getting funding through the typical channels for something as out-of-the-box as his spontaneous-remission study is unlikely. "This is an area of research that is essentially unmapped," he says. "It's not the typical thing to fund." As with other unconventional studies, raising money from private sources is his best bet. "I think that's the only way to do it. I think that's ultimately what it's going to take."

To get the word out, he has given a TEDx talk on the role of the mind in spontaneous remission. He has also started a website, medicineofhopeandpossibility.com, where he writes blog posts and plans to invite people to share their stories—to give other people hope. Providing a space where people can tell their personal positive outcomes represents a shift away from what he calls medicine's focus on what's wrong with people to what's right. "We have a science of disease. So doctors are good at being realistic, but they're not good at giving hope, knowing how to give grounded, realistic hope."

He's a psychiatrist. Helping people tell their stories is what he knows how to do. And these stories, and perhaps ultimately his study, may teach other people about their potential to heal.

10

Annie Salafsky

Saying No to No

*You can't not try, you know? I just can't not because
she deserves everything.*
—Annie Salafsky

Annie Salafsky had no children at breakfast, and by night
she had two. First she gave birth to Daisy. The second baby was Tess,
who was breech, waiting her turn. When the doctor reached in to pull
her out, her toes were the first to feel the air.

Annie felt three kinds of amazement. First, knowing in advance
that she was going to have twins had done little to help her compre-
hend such a multitude. The second stunner was that after a difficult
pregnancy and a few miscarriages before that, her two baby girls were
perfectly fine. Plus, they were just so adorable. All of it was as stagger-
ing as it was mundane.

Annie and her husband, Tom Corwin, stayed home for the next
couple of months taking care of their girls together. Tess was sweet

and rarely cried. While her sister chattered, Tess was quieter and very snuggly. Both girls quickly grew chubby.

The family lives in rural Rochester, Washington. Annie is an organic farmer. She and her business partner grow fifty acres of vegetables, fruit, flowers, and herbs; the produce feeds twelve hundred families annually. Tom is a builder of environmentally sustainable homes. He also raises pigs and chickens, enough to feed the family and have a little left over to barter with a fisherman friend for crab, salmon, and spot prawns.

When the girls were three months old, their grandparents came for a summer feast. It was mid-July and by then the farm was really showing off its bounty. Annie's stepdad, who lived up the road with Annie's mom, made a whole-leaf Caesar salad from feathery Treviso radicchio picked that day. Tom's mom and her boyfriend had just arrived in town for a visit. They all sat at the table, passing the babies around and sipping wine. The lights were off, and the candles were going. They could hear the rush of the nearby river through the open windows.

Tom's mom, Julie, was holding Tess when she became alarmed. "Oh my God, you guys! I think she stopped breathing!" Annie thought she was overreacting. Sure, we have all tiptoed in to check on our children, waiting that extra half-second to see their little chests swell. But it's not as if we're actually afraid. Annie knew that watching to make sure a baby was still breathing was more ritual than prudence.

Even so, they all jumped up. Someone turned on the lights. All six of them stared at Tess. Her little onesie inflated. "Oh, she's fine," someone said. Others chimed in: "That was weird." "Maybe she burped." "It was nothing." Like pundits for a baby channel, they all delivered confident analysis without really knowing anything. Whatever it was, it was over.

Three months later, Annie was playing with Tess on the bed in the sunroom. Lying in her mom's lap, Tess was practicing giggling and general cuteness—she was a natural—while Annie's mom folded baby clothes nearby. Daisy was maybe napping; she's not in this scene.

Tess was smiling and then she wasn't. Her lips started turning blue. Annie had looked away, looked down—and it had started. Tess didn't seem to be breathing. Annie thought instantly of that earlier incident around the table. Her mind touched one thought and flitted to the next like a rock skipping across water: Something was not right. Something was really wrong. Panic.

Annie screamed for her mom, who rushed over. They shook Tess gently and called her name. Her eyes were open but she seemed not to be present. She definitely wasn't breathing. Her face was ghostly.

Thirty seconds later, Tess finally took a breath. Color flooded back into her face, and she came to life again as if someone had found her "on" button.

Annie picked up the phone. She must have called Tom but she remembers talking only to the pediatrician. "Oh, Mom," he told her. "You're just overreacting. I'm sure she's fine." Maybe it was gas, he said.

Annie wasn't reassured at all, and she really wanted to be. "It was this weird moment of transition," Annie tells me. "A lot of the ease I felt as a parent slipped away." Until then, she'd always been able to talk herself down. "'What could happen? Nothing could happen! It's going to be fine! Of course it's fine!' You know, that whole thing," she says. "Suddenly that was just shredded." She realized, "Something can happen and something *will* happen." She was sitting on the back stairs of her house because that was where she could get the best cell reception. She stayed there long after she hung up with the doctor, terrified.

Annie's mom went home in the afternoon and called that night. She had just talked to her ex-husband, Annie's dad, a pediatrician and geneticist. She told him what had happened earlier. He said it sounded like Tess had had a seizure.

A seizure is abnormal activity in the brain. Our neurons use tiny electrical impulses to communicate with one another. During a seizure, too many neurons fire at the same time in a way that overpowers normal signaling, just as a crowd yelling at a stadium can drown out individual conversations. Seizures can lead to bodily injury, brain damage, and sudden death. Sometimes they can be traced to a cause—a brain injury, a tumor, a fever, alcohol or drug withdrawal, or

an infection, such as meningitis. In many cases, though, they're idiopathic, the scientific term for "we have no idea why."

Annie and her father had been estranged for years. Their relationship was in a state of disrepair going back to Annie's childhood. After
high school, Annie headed west to college hoping to ditch her family
and all the unhappiness. Plotting a life that had no resemblance to the
one she'd known in her affluent Chicago suburb, she enrolled at the
Evergreen State College in Olympia, Washington, intent on becoming
a farmer. *See you assholes later!* she thought. In recent years, she and
her father had spoken only two or three times. After her parents di-
vorced, Annie did become closer to her mother, who eventually joined
Annie in Washington.

Before making the call to her dad, Annie had a moment of trepi-
dation. Neither of them had made much of an effort to contact the
other over the years. And now, after so much time, Annie was calling
because she wanted something. It didn't occur to her that the thing
she was asking for was the easiest thing for any father to give, the
thing all parents hate *not* to give: their advice.

She dialed. It was eleven at night in Evanston, Illinois, where her
father lived. He picked up the phone and was all business—not in a
mean way, just in doctor mode. Annie felt deeply grateful for his medical opinion, which she trusted despite her complicated feelings about
their relationship. And maybe she felt some comfort, too, hearing her
father's voice in a difficult hour.

He told her she needed to take Tess to the emergency room.
"Now?" Annie said. It was past nine where they were; Tess and Daisy
had been asleep for hours. He convinced her that she needed to go.
Annie's mom came over to watch Daisy. Annie and Tom plucked Tess
from her crib.

The emergency room at Providence St. Peter Hospital in Olympia
was crowded. While they waited to be seen, Tess was jolly and cooing
under the fluorescent lights. After an hour and a half, they were finally
escorted to an exam room where Tess promptly stopped breathing
again. Annie and Tom yelled for a nurse, who arrived in time to witness the event. It was indeed a seizure.

Then everything shifted. It was as if someone had sounded an alarm that was audible to everyone in the hospital except Annie and Tom, like a dog whistle for doctors. Annie and Tom had just been ignored for almost two hours and now people were streaming in and out of their room. Minutes before, they'd been craving this kind of attention. Now that they had it, they realized how only people in trouble were rewarded in this particular way.

Tess was hooked up to a device that monitored her heartbeats and breathing. She then had two more seizures. Now that she was connected to a machine, her arrested breathing came with a soundtrack, a horrifying, sustained beep that wasn't going to quit until she took in air again. The alarm accompanying their daughter's suffocation did what alarms do, scaring and unsettling its listeners further. Annie and Tom waited.

Once she was breathing again, the doctors examining Tess decided she needed to be transferred to Mary Bridge Children's Hospital in Tacoma, thirty minutes away. Annie and Tom found themselves in an ambulance, its siren shrieking up I-5. Tess was strapped down to the gurney. People were checking her vitals. Annie was blank and numb, a coping strategy she's stuck with over the years. "It doesn't feel like there's a lot of room to be emotional," she says. Tom, a former army tank driver who served in the Gulf War, cries more easily.

When they arrived at the new ER, Annie and Tom were shunted off to the side. A team huddled around Tess, forming a human curtain. They told Annie and Tom what they were doing as they did it, but Annie has no memory of the particulars except when they said they were going to do a spinal tap to check for meningitis.

Annie and Tom were now bit players in their six-month-old's comfort and wellness. The more danger she was in, the further she moved from their grasp, which made practical but not emotional sense. Annie and Tom hugged each other and cried as the needle was driven into Tess's back. "We were wretched by then," says Annie.

They spent two nights, maybe three, at the hospital while Tess underwent more tests, including an MRI. The doctors were looking for the source of Tess's seizures. Through it all she was a champ, rarely crying. She gazed at the halo of strangers' faces hovering above her.

The hospital had a lounge for family members that included a computer. Knowing nothing about seizures, Annie and Tom ventured onto the Internet to find out basic facts. Annie googled "seizures."

An innocent click and she was assaulted by worst-case scenarios and stories of hopelessness. It was an ambush. She remembers her eye catching something saying that 50 percent of kids who have epilepsy develop childhood leukemia. *I'm done!* she thought and shut the computer down. (Like so many things that snag our attention on the Internet, this one, or, at least, Annie's memory of this one, is nonsense. However, some antiepileptic drugs are considered possibly carcinogenic.)

The scary stories had been released into her mind like malware—regardless of whether or not any of it was true or likely in Tess's case. How could she tell? So she walked away feeling afraid of it all. "I was so [insert sound of Annie screaming]!" She had never thought of googling as a reckless act. It would be years before she would search online for information about seizures again.

The doctors didn't find a tumor or meningitis or anything they could trace the seizures to and finally diagnosed Tess with epilepsy. It was a huge relief given the alternatives. The doctors, Annie says, were optimistic about being able to control the seizures with medication.

Tess was prescribed phenobarbital, a highly effective anticonvulsant. While the drug came with some worrying potential side effects, including cognitive difficulties, Tom and Annie were enthusiastic about its great odds of quashing the seizures. So they were exhausted but hopeful when they finally came home from the hospital, pulling into their gravel driveway, which was always puddly with Washington rain.

In the months following her diagnosis, Tess had several more seizures before they got her dosage right.

Then, for the next two years, she was seizure-free.

On most days Tess's family was almost able to forget that she had epilepsy. Not that there wasn't always a gnawing, underlying anxiety, but it was unassertive, like Muzak. They were so religious about giving Tess her medication every day and at the exact same hour that the exercise became rote, their muscle memories sneaking them past emotional trip wires.

Tom and Annie did remain concerned about the cognitive side effects associated with phenobarbital. But the drug was working, so they were "1,000 percent" committed to it. They would just have to stay on top of any related issues so they could work to manage or mitigate them.

With that in mind, they took Tess to see an occupational therapist a couple of months after her diagnosis to get a baseline evaluation. They hadn't noticed that she was having any problems at that point, but the therapist detected that Tess's dexterity was already a little delayed and attributed it to the medication. The OT's observation was upsetting to hear, of course, but it was also clear that the problem wasn't significant.

And Tess was developing so well on other fronts. One of the gauges of her success was Daisy. Always being compared to your twin is one of the great bummers of being one, but for Annie and Tom it was a useful, reassuring tool.

Tess and Daisy would end up hitting all the major milestones as a team. The two girls learned to walk in the same week. They spoke their first words within days of each other. They always had equal weights and were the same height.

And in some ways, Tess was advanced. She had to be told something only once to remember it. She mastered her letters sooner than most babies her age. During one follow-up visit, Tess's neurologist noted in the chart that the twenty-month-old could identify many colors—"even silver"—and recite half the alphabet. Part of Annie was thinking, *Oh my God! She's brilliant!* "Like every parent thinks," she tells me.

When that first summer came around after Tess's diagnosis, the girls were fourteen months old. By then, Annie was at ease enough about her daughter's health that she'd returned to work full-time. She even achieved the fabled and rarely witnessed work–home life balance, that Loch Ness Monster of women's lives.

She'd come home in the evening and immediately load the girls into the off-road stroller to go back up to the fields. They'd cut across the little valley that held their farmhouse, up the road to the lush, green stripes Annie had made in the land. Then the baby girls would help their mom harvest the family's dinner.

Their burgeoning vocabulary was crowded with the names of fruits and vegetables. They'd pick green beans and suck on them. The first concept they mastered was ripeness, which they put into aggressive practice in the raspberry patch. "Ripe! Ripe!" they'd say, plunking the ready fruit into their mouths. For Tess and Daisy, learning to eat real food and learning to talk came in the same package.

The phenobarbital started failing just after Tess's third birthday. One morning she woke up and started the day with a whole series of seizures. And there was Annie again, outside on the phone with the doctor. This time, though, it was Tess's neurologist on the line who told Annie to get Tess to the ER right away.

Tess was put on a higher dose of phenobarbital, but the seizures kept coming. She was back in the ER within about a month. She was having seizures every two hours and they were each lasting thirty seconds. Tess was prescribed a new drug called Trileptal and began weaning off the phenobarbital. The Trileptal seemed to make her angry for the hour after she took it every day. She also started to have trouble falling asleep. But, so far, the new drug seemed to be working. Their hopes were a skyscraper.

Two months later the seizures were back. The doctor upped Tess's Trileptal and decided to delay weaning off the phenobarbital. That was August. By October Tess was having a flurry of three seizures a day, over the course of three days, every month. The Trileptal was abandoned. Next up was Keppra, another anticonvulsant. It seemed to Annie and Tom that the farther they moved down the list, the worse the potential side effects got. Keppra's included sleepiness, coordination problems, joint pain, seizures that are worse than or different from before, dizziness, and suicidal thoughts. They decided to hold off on trying it for the time being, sticking with just the phenobarbital.

As she neared her fourth birthday, Tess was able to feel when a seizure was coming on. And when she did, she would scream "No!" Though she'd been through it many times before, or perhaps because she had, she seemed terrified of what her brain was about to do. But even as she'd protest the onslaught, she would lay herself down and get ready for it, having learned to protect herself from a falling injury.

The seizure would make her quiet. Her eyes would stay open, and she would appear partially aware, seeming to try to focus on her mom or dad at her side. Her hands would usually twitch, but other than that her body wouldn't move.

Seeing Tess this quiet and motionless, you might have believed that she was at peace. Except for the fact that her lips would turn blue. Sometimes she stopped breathing for as long as a minute. And what was happening inside her head looked nothing like stillness. The calm of Tess's appearance masked the squall in her brain.

For Annie and Tom every seizure was traumatic. "All time stops," Annie says. "You're sucked into this black hole. I feel like you go into shock every time it happens. You're still completely functioning. In a way you are weirdly blanked out because it's so overwhelming you have to be so present. That feeling of danger is so immense."

Over time, as Annie and Tom understood more about their daughter's condition, the events became harder to endure. "She's having a stroke basically every time she has one," says Annie, referring to the precarious nature of the seizures.

Every time, they waited to see if she was going to start breathing again. "Every single time!" Annie says, amazed. They could never be sure that she would. "It kind of feels like she's going to die." Saying those words makes Annie cry. She says that it's the first time she's had that thought consciously. Each year, one in one thousand people with epilepsy die suddenly, according to the Epilepsy Foundation.

If you were to average out the frequency of Tess's seizures during that time in their lives, Annie and Tom faced the chance of their daughter's passing away once every three days.

While they continued to see the neurologist, Annie sought out a doctor of naturopathic medicine at Swedish Medical Center in Seattle, two hours away, a medical practitioner with a holistic approach. Annie wanted to make sure she looked everywhere for anything that might help her daughter as a complement to the neurologist's care. "It was a no-stone-unturned thing," she says, echoing the other people in this book. She just kept thinking, *What else can we do?* At the very least, she figured the naturopath might be able to offer guidance on how to keep Tess's liver healthy as she metabolized such hardcore medication.

Annie had started reading a book called *Complementary and Alternative Therapies for Epilepsy*. While she certainly had a natural inclination to wander outside the bounds of traditional medicine— organic farmer and alternative medicine were as natural a pairing as chocolate and peanut butter—she liked the book because it was written by two MDs, one from Harvard, the other from NYU. She was still the daughter of a doctor. She told me that if she'd been the one diagnosed with epilepsy, she would not have gone the conventional route. (She credited an acupuncturist with clearing up her acne, and homeopathy for resolving recurring strep.) But it's different when it's your child. "I didn't feel comfortable taking any risks with her." Plus, she was making the decisions with Tom and his philosophy was very definitely, "Do what our doctors say."

Dr. Dan Labriola, the naturopath, prescribed a number of supplements, including a multivitamin, calcium/magnesium, and digestive enzymes. Annie filled Tess's neurologist in about this other practitioner they were seeing. Recording the information in Tess's chart, the neurologist sounded like she was negotiating a co-parenting arrangement. "Mom would like all of us to work together and she is hoping I am open to naturopathic trials," she wrote.

Soon after she started seeing Dr. Labriola, Tess got some relief from her seizures. Maybe it was a coincidence or maybe she was responding to the additional treatment. Either way: "We were feeling hopeful again," says Annie.

Dr. Labriola suggested they see a colleague of his at Swedish Medical Center, Dr. Marcio A. Sotero de Menezes, a specialist in pediatric neurology and the medical director of the Pediatric Neuroscience Center. Annie and Tom hadn't been all that motivated to get a second opinion before because they liked their current neurologist. And when they'd asked around for recommendations, they'd come up empty. But now that they had Dr. Sotero de Menezes's name, they made an appointment right away. "This was the guy," Annie says. "We were totally excited."

Dr. Sotero de Menezes struck Annie and Tom as very thorough. Their initial appointment with him lasted two hours. He was also sweet and personable. And Dr. Sotero de Menezes had a strategy. Annie says that he thought that a video EEG or electroencephalogram of one of Tess's seizures would help him characterize them better and determine which medication they should try next.

An EEG taps the outer edge of our brains' phone lines, measuring electrical activity from our neurons' chatter. In the test Dr. Sotero de Menezes wanted to do, an EEG is combined with video of the person being monitored, so the outward signs of the seizure can be matched to the brain activity.

Tess would have to be admitted to the hospital. Annie and Tom suggested that they wait until her next seizure cycle began, but they were told that they couldn't book a hospital room that way. (Though Annie granted permission to discuss Tess's case, a spokesperson for Swedish Medical Center declined to comment on Dr. Sotero de Menezes's behalf, citing hospital policy.)

In the meantime Tess turned four. At her party she and Daisy wore dresses and bows in their hair. It was sunny, for once, and all the neighbors and their kids gathered in the Salafsky-Corwin yard. There was quite a bit of noise and commotion and after five months with no seizures, Tess got slammed with a brutal group of them, stress being one of her triggers. Annie took her inside and Tess ended up missing the rest of her party. They sat in the living room while the other kids played outside on the trampoline. Tess had a snack. Annie remembers thinking that the world was passing her daughter by.

Tess was visibly crestfallen to miss her party, but she didn't complain. "It's really crazy, the no-complaining she'll do," says Annie. "She's the most stoic child." If Tess falls and injures herself, she'll run to the other room to hide the fact that she's hurt. If you tell her you're sorry that something happened to her, she'll get angry. At a certain point it occurred to Annie that Tess might be equating feeling bad—when she has a seizure, for example—with being a bad person. "It almost feels like there aren't enough words to talk about what's going on with her," said Annie, who's made a point of asking Tess whether she feels sick rather than bad.

The day came for the video EEG. Tess was checked in to the hospital. Electrodes were glued onto her head, matting down her dark brown curls. They waited.

Nothing. The doctor started reducing her phenobarbital to help bring on a seizure. This seemed like it was doing harm even if it was for a greater good. "It felt terrible. Shocking and terrible," says Annie.

Tess remained hooked up to the electrodes for twenty-four hours a day because the seizures could strike at any second. If she had to go to the bathroom, she could stretch the wires just enough to reach the toilet.

Days went by. The electrodes itched and kept falling off. Her hair became tangled and gloppy with glue. Both Annie and Tom spent the night there with Tess. They asked the doctor again if they could please just come back when Tess was having seizures. No, they could not.

Finally, on the afternoon of her fifth day in her hospital bed, Tess's brain performed: She finally had a seizure. And because she was hooked up to the EEG machine, her brain waves were recorded and translated into zigzagging lines that resemble the lie detector tests from cop shows. In a brain that's functioning normally, the lines form shallow peaks and valleys. On Tess's EEG, the lines exploded into a vicious scribble, row upon row of what appeared like angry-looking, sharp teeth.

Dr. Sotero de Menezes started her on a new drug called Zonegran. They were moving forward again.

But several weeks after she left the hospital, Tess got an antibiotic-resistant staph infection that goes by its acronym, MRSA. It was July and she'd been running around outside when she cut the bottom of her foot on a rock in the driveway. Within twenty-four hours a red line was traveling up her leg like a tide coming in. Most people who get infected with MRSA pick it up in hospitals, and it can be fatal.

As her body fought the infection, she suffered breakthrough seizures—seizures that fall outside and in addition to the usual cycle. After two rounds of heavy-duty antibiotics the deadly bacteria finally surrendered. Tess was okay.

But that autumn Tess came down with pneumonia, and she started seizing nonstop. A seizure would end, then it would start happening again; they'd never been unrelenting like that before. More antibiotics, more hospital visits. That new anticonvulsant, shown to be a dud, was retired.

Then just as she was recovering from the pneumonia, Tess fell apart again. But this time it was into more pieces. Her behavior started disintegrating. She'd always been a sweet, gentle girl. She had danced out the door to preschool. Now she was unruly and stormy with tantrums, refusing to leave the house in the morning. During the lulls she seemed spaced-out. She had terrible headaches, and she seemed to look at people less when she talked to them. She started walking on her tiptoes, and she was obsessed with numbers, letters, and colors. She would talk about the same books constantly and in the same way. At the time Tess was trying yet another anticonvulsant, so it was impossible to sort out if Tess's new problems were side effects or something worse.

But then she lost her toilet training after having managed it for a year. She'd hold in her bowels, sometimes for a week, until she'd have an accident. Her other behavioral issues had been more subtle, murky, difficult for Annie and Tom to be sure of. This one shook their shoulders. They realized, "This is big. This is beyond seizures now."

Annie had wondered about autism before; Tess had always seemed a little different, a little savant-like. But the qualities were always too mild to be concerning. And she was such an affectionate kid, which cut against the typical autism profile. Now Tess's spectrum qualities were much more pronounced. When Annie asked Dr. Sotero de Menezes about it, she said that he attributed her issues to developmental delays from both the medication and the seizures. He said maybe she was a little slow, but that was it. Though Annie was eager to accept what he said—and Tess was still such a loving little girl—she couldn't quite get there. "I was hoping that that was true," she tells me. But she continued to worry. (The Swedish Medical Center spokesperson declined on Dr. Sotero de Menezes's behalf to comment on this aspect of the story as well.)

THERE'S A DEFINITE CONNECTION BETWEEN autism and epilepsy, according to Dr. Orrin Devinsky, the director of NYU Langone's Comprehensive Epilepsy Center who also happens to be one of the authors of Annie's book about complementary therapies for epilepsy. "There's a reciprocal relationship," he tells me. Is one causing the other? "My gut is in some cases, having bad epilepsy hurts the brain to the degree that it does contribute to the autism," he says, adding that what makes it difficult is that there's something wrong with the brain that is causing the epilepsy. So maybe that same problem is leading to autism. "It gets hard to separate them."

Meanwhile, the seizures kept coming. Tess's diagnosis was changed to intractable epilepsy. The picture for her now looked very different. The odds of suppressing her seizures—once on her side—were reversed.

But no one was giving up. How could they? Tess kept trying new anticonvulsants. "Parents agree with plan," Dr. Sotero de Menezes noted in Tess's chart as they trudged ahead.

In the end none of the anticonvulsants they tried worked. Tess remained on the original drug, phenobarbital, because every attempt at weaning her off of it had made things worse. Still the seizures knocked her down every month.

The summer before Tess was supposed to be starting kindergarten, she was evaluated again by an occupational therapist. She'd always impressed her parents with how bright she was. Now she tested two years behind grade level. She was five and unable to form even the precursors to letters.

Annie felt that Tess was getting good care from her new neurologist and her naturopath (they were seeing a new one closer to home), but, at the same time, their ideas seemed somewhat exhausted. It never occurred to her that perhaps there were no solutions. They may not be known, but Annie took it on faith that they existed. She just kept thinking, *I need to do more. I want to do more.*

So she was primed when she heard from her sister who'd heard from her own naturopath that the Specific Carbohydrate Diet could help with seizures.

Annie believed food mattered—it was her life's work. She knew the effect that the right nutrients could have on her crops. Take aphids. Once she had an infestation of the yucky, white crawly bugs, she had to break out an insecticide, which was never that effective. She'd learned that if she made sure she tested her soil before planting and added amendments of macro- and micronutrients, her crops would fare better. The plants' enhanced health made their own natural defenses against pests strong enough to do their job. Annie also realized that she'd get great side effects—parsnips as fat as waffle cones, stalactite-carrots, Swiss chard leaves "the size of a small toddler," in Annie's words.

For Annie, realizing that eating the right food might mitigate Tess's difficulties was like being the pope and having a miracle pointed out to her.

THE SPECIFIC CARBOHYDRATE DIET

The diet was essentially no grains, no starches, no added sugar, no milk, and no family could have been in a better position to make appealing substitutions for those American staples. Of course, restricting her diet meant being different at school—and left out of most celebrations. But at home, away from the taunts of the morsels she wasn't allowed to have, she could feast on the supreme deliciousness of her mom's produce and her dad's farm animals, which became dinner and lunch (leftovers). They would give it a month.

Tess had always picked at pasta and cereal. Now that she was eating eggs with vegetables for breakfast and juices made from berries, carrots, and spinach, Tess started feeling better. Maybe grains and starches had always made her feel bad. Though she didn't say it, "she was sort of like, 'Finally, Stupids!'" says Annie.

One of the highlights became the "snack plate." Annie would pile on some combination of homemade yogurt from their neighbor, carrots, peppers, cucumbers, nuts, raw cookies, dried fruit, and grain-free granola. "That costs more than gold," Annie says of the last item, "but may be worth it."

After two weeks on the new diet Tess's monthly seizure cycle kicked in. This time, Annie noticed that the number of seizures was reduced by a third. The seizures themselves were shorter in duration and less severe. Tess was more awake than she usually was during a seizure. She used to spend the entire three-to-five-day period on the couch moaning, feeling sick, pointing to the spot where her stomach hurt, probably from holding in her bowels. She was still lying on the couch, but she wasn't moaning anymore.

This was something. Annie and Tom thought, *Holy shit.*

IT WAS JUNE WHEN TESS had tested two years behind grade level. In September, after two months on the new diet, Tess started kindergarten. She could now write her letters beautifully. The occupational therapist, Renae Lewandowski, who'd been seeing Tess regularly, was floored by the dramatic change. "It was phenomenal," Lewandowski tells me with Annie's permission.

It wasn't just her handwriting, Tess was making better eye contact, and her bowel movements became normal again. The old, sweet Tess came back.

There's still no known cause of autism and no cure, either. There is, however, a lot of anecdotal evidence and a little bit of controlled scientific evidence that a gluten-free, casein-free diet (gluten and casein are the proteins in wheat and milk, respectively) improves communication and other behavior in some children with autism, according to Dr. Paul Wang, the head of medical research at Autism Speaks, a leading advocacy group.

Maybe the diet was effective because it promoted the right gut bacteria. In 2013, researchers at Caltech reported that mice with autistic-like behavior and leaky guts were lacking in a certain bacterium. After they were fed the bacterium, they became more sociable and their GI issues improved. Autism Speaks is funding further microbiome study.

Even so, Dr. Wang doesn't think diet is going to be the cure. "Diet is important for everybody. It can affect mood, your general cognitive status, but I don't think it is going to have a huge effect on very many kids with autism," he tells me. "It's part of the answer."

As if to prove Dr. Wang's point about the universal relevance of food, Tess's whole family, including the grandparents, adopted her new grain-free, starch-free, milk-free, sugar-free diet. Then it spread to Annie's business partner, Sue Ujcic, and her boyfriend. Everyone started noticing changes. "Your skin is clearing up!" "Oh wow! You lost weight!" They were all feeling more energetic and no one's joints hurt anymore. Tom's asthma improved dramatically. His environmental allergies evaporated. All of which made everyone more inclined to believe that the changes they were seeing in Tess were real—and they were due to all the vegetables, fruits, and farm meats they were sticking to.

"I wanted to stand and scream it on the street corners," says Annie. "Of course, you idiots, it's the food!"

They added together their anecdotal evidence and treated the results like scientific data. It was not, but Annie was starting to have a beef with science. "I just think that we've been convinced that our own observations are suspect. And I don't agree with that," Annie says. She wondered why Tess's neurologists didn't consider food when Tess put it into her body every day.

Annie learned two lessons from seeing Tess improve: one, that it was possible; two, that her own single-mindedness gave them an edge.

Annie started spending entire days in front of the computer reading anything she could find about nutrition and how it might be related to epilepsy and autism. By this point Annie knew all too well how scary their situation was, so she was no longer afraid to search the Internet for information. She plunged into the information democracy online, where all material—proven to be true or not—is presented as equal: Listservs, chat rooms, various medical institution and foundation websites. Without a medical background, she felt like she was the wrong woman for the job, but she was the only volunteer.

Sure, the diet changes seemed to have had a positive effect—if Tess's improvements weren't flukes or attributable to some kind of refracted placebo effect that originated from Annie's resolve—but what gave Annie the idea that she would be able to crack uncontrolled epilepsy when the experts couldn't? "Now that you say that, it does sound kind of conceited," she tells me. "I didn't even realize it was audacious to think I could. I never stopped to think about that part. I'm not saying, like, I'll solve the world's problems. I'll find my answer. So that feels different in a way."

She'd had to figure things out for herself before. In high school, she was swallowed by depression, often not showing up for class. At the same time she believed there had to be a way to climb out of it to find fulfillment. Self-determination wasn't new to her. She'd wanted to play hockey as a child and became the only girl in the league. In grade school she loved to read biographies of great women in history. Annie absorbed their message, that there was a meaningful life to be had if she could just find it. As a teenager, all the adults she knew were highly paid professionals. "It was the eighties, the height of the whole yuppie thing," she says. She looked around and saw that money wasn't delivering on its promise of happiness, including in her own family.

She started questioning, trying to figure out what really counted in life, searching the depths as only divers and teenagers can do. She came up with the idea of farming because the value of food was not debatable. She realized, "This is something we do every day and it's real." She was seventeen.

When Annie decided to become a farmer, it was before chicken coops were chic and before people younger than Don Rickles did their own pickling. She started working in the fields the summer after her freshman year of college, and she was as happy as she was filthy. The physical labor took her on a vacation from her own mind, away from all her existential angst.

She was twenty-four when she went into business with Sue Ujcic. The act of farming has made them close friends. "For ten hours a day, you're out there. Boring, boring. So what do you do? You just talk talk talk and basically therapize each other all day." Working with her hands, being her own boss, eating well, all of it continues to be restorative for Annie.

It was Annie's independent flair that grabbed Tom the night they met at a mutual friend's wedding. "I could tell she was a bit—this might sound silly—iconoclastic. I could see that in her," Tom tells me. "She lived here by herself," he says, referring to the worn and charming house where I've spent a couple of days with their family. "She was a farmer. It wasn't necessarily what everyone was saying you should be doing. She was going for it." Tom remembers thinking, *That's really awesome! You're rad. I would like to know you.*

Annie's dark, curly hair was longer then, but Tom had the same buzz cut and sideburns. She wore lipstick, which she doesn't bother with much these days. It had been a year since she'd had a terrible breakup, and she had finally recovered. "It was this really magical, unencumbered, perfect time," she says of that night. Tom ended up back at Annie's house. They kissed in the kitchen.

"Thanks for asking me that question," Tom says of my inquiring about how they met. "I love . . . It was good times," he says. "We were very . . ." says Annie, trailing off. "We had fun back in the day."

When Tess got sick, the two of them were natural allies. At first, Annie had reflexively shut down. Tom made a point of saying to her that he was an equal partner. "I'm here, too. Let's do this together," he said. He would tell Annie to go lie down and take a break. "He was trying to take care of me, too," she says. Under this new stress, they collapsed into each other rather than falling away.

As Annie got deeper into her quest to figure out how to help Tess, though, there was less time for Tom, less time for anything else. After the kids were in bed Annie would spend the evenings reading. The two of them used to play Scrabble, look at magazines, talk. Over time, Tom became another husband somewhat cuckolded by illness.

By then, Annie had shifted tactics from random Internet searches to reading books, which felt more legit and had always been her support. She would dog-ear so many pages that the books almost looked like their upper-right corner had been lopped off. "Mom! More books!" Daisy would yell, seeing the mail truck rumble up their driveway.

A book by a Cleveland dentist who died in 1948 led Annie to want to try another experiment with food. Curious why crowded, crooked teeth seemed to be becoming more common, Weston A. Price studied isolated, traditional populations and their diets. He concluded that the unmodern menu, packed with whole fruits, vegetables, and animal products, supplied as much as ten times the nutrients as the carte du jour. Price argued that the flawed smiles he saw on people who'd abandoned traditional diets were marks of physical degeneration brought on by vitamin and mineral deficiencies. He was like a proto–Terry Wahls, calling for a more nutrient-dense diet.

Annie and Tom thought one way they could amp up Tess's nutrition and animal fat consumption would be to make fresh bone broths from the pigs Tom butchered. Annie also started giving her fermented foods, raw, aged cheeses, and sausages.

This time, they didn't notice an improvement in Tess.

Tom started to wonder if maybe his wife was letting Tess's epilepsy control too much of her life, that it was taking up too much of her time. In fact, it was taking up all of her time, but was that too much? What's too much?

Others who cared about Annie questioned what she was actually doing, if she was helping Tess at all. A good friend of Annie's sat her down. She told Annie that she had a friend who worked with autistic kids and that it seemed like Annie needed to work on embracing Tess for who she was. Annie listened. She appeared to be taking her friend's words to heart. But the whole time she was thinking, *Shut up. Shut up. Shut up.*

Then it was Tom's turn. "Maybe we should just accept that this is how she is," he said. "And not try and change her constantly." It was an understandable argument and it hit Annie harder coming from Tom. She nodded. What was going through her mind? "I pretended I agreed and then I just chucked it," she says.

"I mean, there is probably a grain of truth in that," Annie says, referring to the value of acceptance. After all, Tess had at least one and possibly two conditions that had no known cures. "At the same time," Annie says, "she's sick. If she had a broken leg, you wouldn't sit and tell me not to fix it."

Over time, the frequency and intensity of Tess's seizures reverted back to how they'd been before she'd adopted the Specific Carbohydrate Diet. She held on to the gains she made on the autism front, but the epilepsy was a monster.

Annie got back to work. Two books argued that the broth and other new dietary additions might be hurting Tess. Annie told Tom that they were going to have to make another change. "Okay, now my research says she shouldn't eat bone broth. Or fermented foods. And grapes are bad for her," Annie told him. "He was like, 'Fuck you. What is this based on?'" Annie was a little sheepish when she answered him. "I just know?"

Annie was used to making quick decisions whenever problems arose on the farm, which was all the time. A mouse got stuck in a hose. The tractor won't start. She'd built up a lot of confidence in her own instincts.

Tom had been completely supportive before—especially since the first diet change had seemed to work so well. But this was starting to feel absurd. "When you don't know, you shouldn't dabble, because you don't know," he argued.

In the end, he agreed to make the change because he didn't see the harm, but the tension didn't quickly defuse. They'd made such a good team before, the two of them. Now they were still on the same side, but Tom found himself playing a different position. While she played offense, he was trying to rein her in.

Her dad, with whom she was speaking more frequently, would ask, "How can you know any of it is true? Have you run double-blind tests?" Annie used to think, "Oh, whatever. What harm could any of it do? It's just food."

But with the bone-broth reversal she came to think that she could do harm. "I was getting really confused about all of this," she says.

Bone broths and many of the other foods Tess had been eating were rich in glutamate, which is an excitatory neurotransmitter, meaning it tells neurons to fire—delivering messages from cell to cell. So it was not unreasonable to assume that glutamate from food might trigger Tess's excitable neurons. NYU's Dr. Devinsky, who is not affiliated with Tess's case, tells me that the effect of eating glutamate is uncertain but that it is unlikely that it's a major factor. The question is how glutamate you eat could infiltrate the brain.

The blood brings oxygen to the brain, but most other molecules are kept out by a membrane called the blood-brain barrier. It screens out interlopers, a bit like the lining of the intestinal walls.

The blood-brain barrier, however, can become compromised. Like a hyper-permeable gut lining, it can start letting through harmful materials. In fact, a growing body of evidence suggests that a disrupted blood-brain barrier may "precede, accelerate, or contribute to" neurodegenerative disorders including epilepsy, ALS, Alzheimer's, and MS, according to the authors of a 2008 review in *Neuron*.

Annie says that she saw some improvement in Tess's seizures after limiting her intake of glutamate-rich foods. And, going forward, she vowed to be less willy-nilly about experimentation. She would have the naturopath vet an idea first.

Annie says that she would tell the neurologist, Dr. Sotero de Menezes, about whatever they were trying at home, she says—whether it was a new diet or supplements—but he didn't have anything to say about it. He'd listen silently until she was done talking, Annie says, then move on with the conversation. Once, though, his nurse did follow up with a conversation about another diet they might consider. After a couple of years with Dr. Sotero de Menezes, the family returned Tess to the care of her original neurologist.

At one point the naturopath suggested that Tess try medical marijuana, which other kids with uncontrolled epilepsy had reportedly had luck with. (It is now legal for children to be given medical marijuana in Washington State.) I spoke to Annie after Tess started it. "It's fucking working," she said. She was afraid to get too excited, but the rate of Tess's seizures had plummeted 75 percent.

MEDICAL MARIJUANA

Annie says that Tess's doctor was supportive of their use of medical marijuana but, because she was unfamiliar with it, did not offer guidance. (The spokesperson at Mary Bridge Children's Hospital did not respond to multiple messages seeking comment on this and other aspects of Tess's care, though Annie granted permission.)

As thrilling as Tess's progress was, Annie was disturbed by the other effect of the cannabis. The strain Tess was taking was 40 percent THC (tetrahydrocannabinol), the psychoactive component of marijuana, and she definitely seemed a little high on it—giggly and hungry. So Annie and Tom tried switching her to a strain that was pure cannabidiol or CBD, a non-psychoactive chemical in marijuana. Tess's seizures exploded. She had more seizures than she'd ever had and some lasted an hour. She gagged and vomited. When they went back to the original variety, it didn't work, and they abandoned it.

The effect of cannabis on treatment-resistant epilepsy is still not well understood, and neither are its risks. NYU's Dr. Devinsky, who studies the drug's effect on epilepsy, says that what *is* known about marijuana should give everyone pause. "I can tell you that the cannabidiol [in marijuana] almost certainly has drug interactions that are important," he says. And the other main ingredient in marijuana, THC, can cause a number of problems in adolescents including addiction, memory problems, and higher rates of psychiatric disorders such as schizophrenia, he says.

Dr. Devinsky led a team that completed a study of cannabidiol. The results, published in *The Lancet Neurology* in 2016, hold promise. Seizures were reduced by more than a third in the adults and children who completed the trial, all of whom had particularly tough cases of treatment-resistant epilepsy. But since there was no control group that was given a placebo, the numbers are on shaky ground.

Until there's more study, Dr. Devinsky urges parents to put on the brakes, but he is also sympathetic. He knows how desperate they are. "I get it," he says. "I take care of these parents. I see them all day long. I'm on their side. We just have to find a middle ground."

I MEET TESS WHEN SHE is about to turn eight. She looks me in the eye and says hello. She is delightful. Daisy, no slouch, makes me an egg cream with real vanilla extract and stevia drops. If Tess is on the spectrum, she is clearly on the lighter end. She slides onto her mom's lap seamlessly, as if there were no transition from standing to sitting. When she talks to her dad, she touches his cheek. When you see how loving and patient he is with her, it seems clear that the reason he made the case to his wife that they needed to accept Tess for who she was, was because he already had.

When I return to the house the next morning, low clouds have settled on the grass in their valley like cotton balls snagged on Velcro. Inside, the family seems like every other family, caught up in the where-are-my-shoes, here-is-your-lunch bustle before school. They take a break from the whirl to sit together at the table for breakfast. Tom makes an egg, onion, and ham scramble and Annie produces an olive-green juice by smithereening carrots, celery, apples, and spinach in the blender. Tess asks me what I think of my juice and the color of the straw she's picked out for me. Soon her aide, who is with Tess at school in case she has a seizure, arrives—she commutes one minute from the yurt she and her fiancé rent on the property. She whisks both girls to school.

Later that evening I get to see Tess at work. She is a fervent artist. Her paintings, including lovely abstract watercolors, veneer the fridge and one entire wall of her bedroom. She is the same girl who knew her colors early on. She is so enthusiastic, pressing so hard, that the soothing sound of her rubbing a colored pencil on paper is repeatedly interrupted by the sound of a snapping twig: She keeps breaking her pencil tips. Daisy, who seems to have embraced an older-sister role with her twin, admonishes her not to be a spendthrift with her new gold-colored pencil.

If Tess's commitment to coloring has something to do with autism spectrum disorder, it doesn't seem like a bad thing. In fact, it seems like an exciting part of who she is.

Tess has kept academic pace with Daisy. The two are in the same class at the local private school. In the afternoons Tess takes horseback riding and gymnastics. But she does seem younger. She has her own special swing in the living room, crafted out of a hammock; it is calming for her.

The two girls are close. They have smooshed their beds up against each other so they can hold hands while they sleep.

Tess's seizures are now coming at night. When she feels one approaching, she screams, "Seizure!" and sits up in bed. Either Annie or Tom race into her room to try to talk her through it, get her to take a breath. When she does inhale, the event ends. After a seizure Annie goes back to bed but never to sleep. Her heart banging away, she waits for her daughter to scream again. Every month, for five nights in a row, Tess has between one and three seizures a night.

Recently Tom started setting up a cot next to Tess's bed once the monthly cycle of seizures starts. That way, he can be right beside her when a seizure strikes. And, unlike Annie, he's able to quiet his anxiety enough to fall asleep afterward, a skill he learned in the army.

Annie still credits food for the improvements in Tess's autism qualities. And even if it isn't the reason, there is at least no downside, she figures. "She has great eating habits. At the very least, she's going to be one hell of a healthy girl."

It is at their table that I eat some of the best-tasting food of my life. We have roast chicken one night. Though the preparation is familiar, the bird—raised by Tom—is more chickeny, more itself. If this once-feathered creature were a man, you'd describe him as having come into his own.

Then Tom offered me bacon. I don't want to say that it changed my life, but it changed my life. When it hit my tongue, I was filled with dread for when the bite would be over.

Tom had sliced it from a slab of pig that was dangling over our heads from the kitchen ceiling, curing as we spoke. It was difficult to ignore that it was hanging there, like mistletoe. Bacon mistletoe.

ANNIE'S DRIVE TO FIND HELP for Tess is as robust as ever. Next up, a type of helminth, and possibly the ketogenic diet, an extreme, fat-heavy plan that has helped some children with epilepsy. She wonders what a fecal transplant might do for Tess on the basis of emerging research about the link between our microbiomes and so many diseases, though not necessarily epilepsy. (The Specific Carbohydrate Diet that Tess stuck to was predicated on restoring balance to gut bacteria.) "I'll just keep going," she says. "I feel like a wolverine or something. I can't stop!"

Does she feel like there is a chance that she might not ever reach the answer? She acknowledges that there is. "It's not a good feeling," she tells me. And then in almost the same breath she says, "I feel like I'm getting close."

"You can't not try, you know? I just can't not because she deserves everything," she says. Annie has been at this for years and has seen only a small difference in Tess. It has been grueling and isolating and devastating. The tests, the books, the appointments, the supplements add up to a lot of money. "Financially, it's taken all we had," Annie says.

I ask her how it is that she doesn't get discouraged. Annie has a simple answer. "She's not better yet."

POSTSCRIPT: AS TIME WENT ON, Tess's seizures became dramatically worse. By the fall of 2014, they were coming fifteen times a day, every day. Some of them lasted for an hour. And the longer a seizure lasts, the more likely it is to cause brain damage. Annie, being Annie, wouldn't give in. Desperate and crying, she called her sister-in-law, Julie Segre, a senior investigator at the NIH's National Human Genome Research Institute. (It was from Segre that I first heard about Annie's quest, when I interviewed her about the microbiome.) Annie thought that maybe Segre could point them to someone who had an idea of what to do. Segre told Annie: "I want to help. Let me brainstorm."

Segre first went to her computer and network of friends and tried to find out as much as possible about state-of-the-art therapy, she tells me. She talked to a friend of hers from yoga class whose sister is a researcher studying ketogenic diets. She called another friend, a doctor, who looped in her neurologist husband. He recommended a Seattle neurologist he'd trained with, a doctor he said was both personally kind and professionally very astute and careful.

Dr. James Owens is a pediatric neurologist and epilepsy specialist at Seattle Children's Hospital. Because he is the program director for the child neurology residency program at the University of Washington as well as an associate professor of neurology, he doesn't see many patients, especially new ones. When Segre's friend's husband contacted him about Tess, Dr. Owens emailed his scheduler about finding her an appointment.

It took almost two months, but Tess finally saw him. Dr. Owens suggested they get an up-to-date picture of Tess's brain, so he sent her for an MRI. Annie, Tom, and Tess were still in the car, driving home after getting the scan done, when Dr. Owens called. He said that Tess appeared to have a benign tumor the size of a robin's egg; it was most likely the cause of her seizures.

It had been there all along. In fact, it was visible on that first MRI Tess had had as a baby, the only other time she'd gotten one. The tumor in that earlier image is very small and subtle, though, something that would be hard for any neuroradiologist to see without knowing it's there, says Dr. Owens, who spoke to me with Annie's permission.

Dr. Owens says that for patients with uncontrolled epilepsy

and a normal MRI, repeating the image study at regular intervals—perhaps in six months to a year for infants and very small children—is the standard of care for epilepsy. Annie says that Tess's two previous neurologists never suggested she get another MRI. (I reached out to both of their hospitals again but was not able to get comments.)

Dr. Owens says that the discovery of the tumor is partly the benefit of a second opinion. "Sometimes it's about starting with fresh eyes."

IN EARLY SPRING 2016, TESS underwent surgery and the tumor was removed. In Annie's email to me afterward I counted eight exclamation points.

As of this writing, it's too early to know what the effect will be. Dr. Owens won't attempt to taper her antiseizure medication for a couple of months. But Annie, Tom, Daisy, and Tess have good reason to be hopeful. Almost all epileptic children who have that particular kind of tumor successfully removed walk away seizure-free.

11

The Science of Hope

___

Agency vs. Learned Helplessness

IN THE 1960S AT THE UNIVERSITY OF PENNSYLVANIA, A COUPLE of graduate students conducted a series of experiments that to this day offers one of the best possible explanations for why some people keep trying while others don't. These were the experiments Angela Duckworth described as the basis for our understanding of why having control matters so much.

In one experiment, three groups of dogs were put in cages with their heads held in place by two panels. The dogs in the first group received intermittent shocks to their hind feet. They were able to stop the current by pressing one of the panels with their heads. The dogs in the second group received shocks but were powerless to do anything about them—their panels didn't function. The third group, which was the control, didn't get any shocks.

The next day the dogs were placed in boxes that were divided into two sections by a low wall. All three groups received shocks through the floor, but the dogs could escape the unpleasant sensation by jumping to the other side of the box. Almost all of the dogs that had been able to turn off the shocks the day before quickly leapt over the barrier to relief. So did those in the control group who'd never been shocked. And what about the poor dogs who had had no control over their situation the day before? Two-thirds of them made no effort to escape the new shocks.

The young researchers, Martin Seligman and Steven Maier, proposed that the dogs in the first group kept trying to escape the shocks on day two because the animals understood that they had some control over their circumstances. The dogs in the second group had evidently learned that they had no control. And if you are powerless to change your situation, why bother trying to do so? The results have been repeated in many other kinds of animals and in college students.

The phenomenon became known as learned helplessness, and it suggested that having an experience of control was an important factor in the drive to keep trying. On the flip side, a lack of control was related not only to giving up but to depression, as Angela Duckworth, the Penn psychologist, told us. Feeling hopeless is one of the main symptoms of the mood disorder.

How to explain the people in these pages who kept trying? Isn't a diagnosis of an incurable disease the very definition of not having control?

"I wouldn't agree with that," says Steven Maier, who coauthored the dog studies as a graduate student and is now director of the Center for Neuroscience at the University of Colorado at Boulder. "Let's take something even more extreme. Let's say your spouse dies," he says. "Obviously no one believes they have control over that in a direct way. But people do differ in the degree to which they believe they have control over the negative circumstance that has left them in. Some people feel, 'This is really bad. I'm lonely now, but I don't have to be lonely forever. I can join a church group and meet people.' Whereas other people say, 'Oh, there's nothing I can do.' Even in the face of something that looks uncontrollable people differ dramatically in their belief. Some people who get a diagnosis of a disease—let's say cancer. Some people believe, 'Well, I can't will my cancer away so of course I don't have that kind of control, but I can get on the Web and I can look to see if there are any clinical trials going on in my area with new drugs.' So some people believe there are things they can do," he says. "That is a belief in control. That's why they're continuing to try."

Okay, so how do you come by that kind of something-I-can-do belief that Maier's talking about? His own later research offers a possible answer.

He subjected adolescent rats to a scenario of shock and control similar to the dog test. One group of rats got little shocks to the tail but could make them stop by turning a wheel. The second group had no means of turning off the shocks. Maier points out that the shocks did not cause pain—they were more annoying than anything else.

By studying rats, an animal that doesn't live very long, Maier was able to track them for their entire life span. And what he observed was that the young rats that had an experience of control were affected by it *for the rest of their lives*. The early incident—they were teenagers in rat years—inoculated them against helplessness later.

Can we conclude, then, that the belief that it was worth trying came from having overcome that difficult circumstance early on? "Possibly," Maier tells me. But he's cautious. "There's no definitive way to answer that. This kind of research never can tell you for sure in an individual instance whether that really was it or not. But yes, the evidence suggests that an experience of control over a really bad outcome at time one will inoculate you against the debilitating effects of something that's not controllable at a later time, too."

Learning that you have some control sounds like a form of hope. "There are people who would say that," he says. "I'm a rat and mouse guy so I'm not going to talk about hope in a rodent. I don't know what goes on in their consciousness or even if they have any."

Maier has since been able to locate the precise circuit in the rat brain that reacts to the early experience of behavioral control. That circuit activates other circuits, triggering the rat's instinct to protect itself from harm. "It's got nothing to do with consciousness. It's got nothing to do with feelings. It's specific brain circuits."

Much hinges on when the early experience occurs. "In rodents—this is rodents now, right?—in rodents, experiences of control during adolescence are particularly potent because the brain systems involved in this process are still plastic and not fully formed," says Maier. How you translate that to human ages is hard to say, he tells me. "I would say you're going to get these prolonged effects as long as these connections are not fully formed." The human brain continues to develop into our twenties. Until then it's especially sensitive to experience. Afterward, it remains plastic—that's how we learn—but the window for fundamental changes has closed. It's the difference between new construction and a renovation.

Angela Duckworth is less restrained about the significance of Maier's rat study. She warns that it's one experiment but calls the work "totally mind-blowing." She tells me, "They followed these rats until they were adults and they couldn't make the rats helpless! He came and gave this talk in this dusty lecture hall at Penn seven years ago. I was like, 'Dude, I'm getting on a plane and flying to Colorado to see you because, stop the presses, this is huge!'"

The idea of being *inoculated for life* against a feeling is incredible. So is the suggestion that possessing a quality as important and complex as hope could basically come down to flipping a switch. The circuit is possibly the link between the personal experiences Duckworth was talking about earlier and the future expectation that you can do something to change your situation.

I want to know how we can activate this circuit without going through trauma, and this is exactly what Maier is working on. He's been able to activate the right pathways chemically, by putting drugs directly on the neurons in a rat's brain. "It reproduces all of the protective effects of behavioral control," he says. So just like the rat that's able to turn off a shock by turning a wheel, this rat appears to be protected against feeling helpless. The difference is, this second rat, with drugs on his neurons, didn't have to overcome shocks. He tells me, "That is not yet obviously ready for the clinic because you're not going to do that to a person. But it is a proof of principle, right? If we could figure out a way that you could turn on those circuits in a human, that ought to be therapeutic."

Maier thinks talk therapy might also be able to do the job of activating these key pathways in the brain. "We think the therapies that are effective, like cognitive behavioral therapy, in fact do turn on these exact circuits. Human neuroimaging, [such as functional MRI], tends to support that. We haven't proved that. The hypothesis at this point is that some talk therapies may tap into these same circuits.

"I'm a neurobiologist"—meaning he studies the structure and function of the nervous system cells—"but I'm a fan of talk therapies," he says. "I think they work because they affect the brain, not because it's voodoo or something. You are your brain and so this is all about specific brain circuits and how they operate."

He explains why cognitive behavioral therapy might work. "If you think about cognitive behavior therapy, what's it teaching people? That they have control over their negative emotions. Because it's giving you the tools to make them less bad, to reevaluate them. That's telling you, 'Hey, you have some control over this. You're not just a passive recipient of these things.'"

GETTING BACK TO THE FIRST experiment in this chapter, with the dogs: Some of them didn't need the experience of control to make them try to escape round two of shocks. They were determined to escape the shocks even though they hadn't had the experience in the lab of overcoming a difficult event, although it's impossible to know what happened to them before they were adopted for research. As Duckworth describes it, "They were like, 'Fuck this! I'm going to keep jumping over the wall, seeing what I can do.'" This sounded to me like Jamie, not only because of the language.

To Maier, those dogs' resilience doesn't necessarily mean that they were just born that way. "It's certainly not impossible that there are genetic differences in predispositions toward acting on your environment. But certainly your early experiences would affect that, too. All kinds of factors could interact in very complicated ways to determine how you respond to bad things that occur in your environment." As an example, he says that the adult behavior of a rodent is affected by its position in the uterus relative to the others in the litter. Female mouse fetuses who develop adjacent to males tend to have elevated testosterone levels—and more aggressive behavior as adults—than females who didn't have male neighbors in the womb.

I ask Maier what he makes of the fact that most of the main people in this book overcame difficult circumstances when they were young. "You can never explain an individual," he says. "Science doesn't operate that way. It's about groups and about tendencies. Yeah, we know that some people are quite resilient relative to others and will never give up. The animal research suggests the kinds of experiences they may have had earlier in life that lead to this persistence. But you can't discount genetics and epigenetics"—the turning on and off of genes—"and all kinds of subtle things. You never know why any given individual—not from science anyway—is the way they are. It's complicated interactions of genetics and experiences. All kinds of things beginning before birth.

"What makes you as an adult you is a horrendously complicated issue involving everything and so I can't make anything out of six people except that they're highly praiseworthy. At some point science breaks down and it's almost not a scientific issue. How to understand this? How do you understand Joan of Arc, or any of the individuals who are just outstanding? What made them that way? Well, everything made them that way."

12

Trusting Her Son

Amy and Jaxon Chan Take On ADHD with Diet

I didn't want to change my mind.
I wanted to keep how fast my brain moves.
—JAXON CHAN

WHAT DOES A MOTHER DO WITH A CHILD DIAGNOSED WITH ADHD?

When Jaxon was a third grader, the seat of his chair seemed to be rigged with an invisible spring. He was a student at a private, Mandarin immersion school in California. He went through the day like a jack-in-the-box with no lid, popping up onto his feet ten times an hour. He wanted a drink of water. He had to go to the bathroom. He forgot his book in his locker. He needed to grab a pencil from his backpack. Then he needed to sharpen it. He needed his homework, his eraser, his sweatshirt. And he very much needed to chat with his buddies even though they were trying to pay attention to what the teacher was saying.

"He was kind of crazy," says his good friend Collin. "He was kind of like hyperactive and stuff." Kai, another buddy, who lives around the corner from Jaxon, remembers that the teacher would let Jaxon run around. According to Kai, she understood that he had problems. "He would actually, like, go outside the classroom."

Jaxon used to get really, really mad at his friends if they ever disagreed with him. "He thinks he's right?" Kai says, using the unintentional interrogative. And he would just start yelling. "Sometimes Jaxon would, like, punch people," says Collin. And when he got bad grades, he wanted to die. He was nine years old, and he hated himself.

I meet Jaxon and his friends when they're in fifth grade. Though it's two years after the fact, Jaxon can still remember how terrified he was that he'd have to repeat third grade. The memory comes out present-tense fresh. "I have really good friends in my grade and if I get held back that would make life so much harder and there would be kids that were so much younger than me and it wouldn't feel right and I'd have to go through the grade all over again," Jaxon says, his sentence running on with the persistence of worry.

It wasn't that he couldn't keep up with the academics. Jaxon was obviously bright. "He's kind of like scientific-y," Collin says. In fact, Jaxon explains the origin of the universe to me: "There were just these planets of, like, matter and antimatter floating in this void and then one day a couple of them, like, crash really hard."

The trouble came when he had to convert the swirling intelligence in his head into words on a page, as if there were a barricade between his brain and the hand holding his pencil. So he would simply avoid that route altogether. "I just stood up and walked around because I didn't want to do it. And then I would stall until the school day was over." He sometimes handed in blank sheets of paper.

Jaxon was getting in trouble all the time, and he took it hard. The way that the teachers spoke to him was disturbing. "It feels like they purposely try to make you feel insecure and whatnot," he says. "The way they say it is just gut-wrenching."

Every day, after tussling through school, he went home to be confronted with yet another adversary. Homework. Not only were there reading and writing assignments in English and Chinese, but math problems came in both flavors, too. He would often take a seat at a table next to the living-room window. It was an expanse of glass open to the spangled Pacific in the distance until the fog puffed in like a daily fumigation.

The standoff between boy and work would begin. The struggle to focus was excruciating. Every unproductive minute would intensify the pain. Jaxon would surrender, dissolving into a watery meltdown. Then he'd retreat to his bedroom to try to calm down. Then he'd sneak videogames or read comic books. The whole shebang could last three hours.

It's not that Jaxon lacked the will to get it done, his mother, Amy Chan, says. "It genuinely seemed like a mental barrier that was as strong as any physical wall that he simply could not overcome."

Having difficulty in school wasn't new. When he was first learning to read, he fell behind quickly. Amy took him to a reading specialist to try to understand what was going on. Jaxon was diagnosed with a learning disability in reading, which Amy would spend the next few years working with him to overcome. She figured Jaxon's homework trouble was related to his reading issues and that she would just need to help him through it as she'd always done. Though she was working full-time as a lawyer, Amy's hours started early and wrapped up in time for her to take care of the kids in the afternoons.

She tried having Jaxon listen to music on an iPod while he worked. She tried giving him chewing gum. She tried going to cafés and giving him a snack while he was studying. She tried putting something weighted on his shoulders, wrapping his stuffed animals in one of her scarves and hanging the silken hammocks from his neck—"Can't remember where we got THAT idea!"

They tried sitting at a desk at the school library, at the public library, at Starbucks, home at the dinner table, at the coffee table, on the floor. His father, Daniel, whom Jaxon adores, tried sitting right next to his son for as long as it took. That actually worked pretty well, but Daniel was often traveling for business. (Daniel is not his real name. Chan is also not Jaxon's or his father's last name.)

Everyone was bruised by the daily ordeal. Trying to get Jaxon through his homework felt to Amy like pulling "a ten-ton boulder up a double black diamond slope while an entire village was trying to slide it downhill," she wrote to me in an email. "Battle-weary and completely and utterly spent thereafter, leaving nothing emotionally, mentally, or physically to give to my daughter . . . and racked with guilt."

The tension and weariness fed on each other. Wars raged nightly. As for his little sister, Anderson, she was obviously in cahoots with her mother. "Both of them purposefully got mad at me," Jaxon says.

Amy would seek out peace in her bedroom—only Jaxon would be right on her tail. She'd lock the door. So he would lift the lever up and down, up and down, the sound of which was its own bombardment.

He was never not fighting, whether it was with people or schoolwork. And it was exhausting. Come Saturday, he'd plead with his mom for a "pajama day" so he could lie in bed and play videogames until dinner.

As third grade progressed, Jaxon was invited to join a boys' group that met during lunch in the counselor's office to talk about self-regulation strategies. When Amy emailed the teacher asking how progress would be measured, she responded that it wasn't that structured. Amy wrote back: No, thank you, then. Jaxon needed his lunch-period downtime. She thought the school was biased against spirited boys and didn't know how to handle them. She imagined Jaxon's teacher getting her response and drumming her fingers on the table. (The headmaster declined on behalf of his staff to comment for this story, citing a school privacy policy.)

Finally the school called Jaxon's parents in for a sit-down. The meeting took place in the counselor's office, but Amy and Daniel felt as if they'd been called to the principal's. They walked in and, as they recall, were met by the school counselor, the reading specialist, the learning specialist, Jaxon's English teacher, and his Chinese teacher. They were all there to talk about the slight third grader who'd just turned ten. They took seats around a coffee table. Throats were cleared. It was all very awkward—perhaps because Jaxon's dad was vice chair of the board of trustees.

Jaxon's English teacher would end up doing most of the talking, but before she could start, Amy needed to know something right away. Were they there because Jaxon was going to be held back? She'd been in as much of a panic as her son about his chances of advancing to fourth grade. She had spun out the horrible ways it would affect him. She worried that it would derail him from college and graduate school and, as a result, leave him financially insecure.

No, Jaxon was not going to be held back, the school counselor told Amy. But the teachers had more to say. "He's not performing at the level that's reflecting our assessment of his natural intelligence," Amy remembers their saying. "He is just so much smarter than the quality of the work he is providing. He is so much smarter than a typical kid who gets up ten times in a session of class."

Previous teachers had mentioned that he got up a lot, but they'd been able to handle it—giving him a stick of gum or having him sit on a ball, for example, typical strategies for that kind of child, says Daniel. While he and Amy were certainly aware that Jaxon was a boisterous boy and that getting him to focus on homework was what it was, this was the first time they were hearing that his disruptions in class were extreme, about the incessant trips to the locker, the water fountain, the bathroom.

It was the unarticulated message the group delivered that morning that hit harder. "When I walked into that meeting, that visual of all of them there communicated the severity of what message they were trying to deliver. They had to make a cost-benefit analysis of taking both teachers away from all forty kids to talk to you about one kid." The message Amy and Daniel received was this: Jaxon was a problem for the teachers that needed to be fixed. And the school was running out of patience.

Amy and Daniel say that the school representatives asked them to get Jaxon tested, including having his vision and eye-tracking checked, and asked for permission to do their own assessments. "Fine," Amy said, feeling the weight of them bearing down on her. "Assess away."

The school referred Jaxon to an educational psychologist who gave him the diagnosis of ADHD: attention deficit/hyperactivity disorder.

Children with ADHD tend to be extremely active and have trouble focusing or controlling their behavior or any combination of the above.

Though they hadn't suspected ADHD, Amy and Daniel weren't surprised by the diagnosis, either. They realized that they were a bit ADHD themselves. On Amy's own kindergarten report card, her teacher had written, "Has natural intelligence, but talks too much and can't sit still." Daniel used to get "improvement needed" on his report cards. "That was the F in public elementary school," he says. Maybe that's another reason—in addition to the reading disability they thought was the thing making homework hard—why they hadn't recognized the ADHD themselves: Jaxon's behavior resembled their normal. Amy was disappointed that she'd passed her issues on to her son.

The educational psychologist, who was given permission to speak about Jaxon but declined to comment, told Amy and Daniel that stimulants like Ritalin that were used to treat ADHD were safe and had been around a long time, according to Amy. They'd need to get a prescription from Jaxon's pediatrician.

Amy felt that she was being pressured to medicate Jaxon. "He was very careful with the choice of his words," says Daniel. "What he said was, 'You can try a lot of different things and people have had varying degrees of success, but the only method that we know for sure that works is medication,'" says Daniel. Amy heard the psychologist differently. "He flat-out said, 'Meds are the only way to go.'"

Listening through her own emotional filter, Amy traced the pressure she was feeling to medicate Jaxon through the psychologist to the school. She was afraid that the school was trying to label her son a problem and would eventually counsel him out—recommend he transfer, or force him to. (Though Amy and Daniel granted permission, the headmaster declined to comment on this and all aspects of the story due to school policy.)

The truth was Amy had had it, too. Jaxon had been getting 60s on his exams; she didn't want another tarnished year on his record. And while she and Daniel resented the pressure for him to perform perfectly, they weren't immune to it. At the school, they were surrounded

by high-achieving parents who compared and measured the performance of their children against one another, says Daniel. Is your kid
going to go to Stanford? Is your kid going to go to Harvard? At a birthday party, one parent talked about meeting the director of admissions
at MIT. His daughter was in kindergarten. "My GPA was 2.91 out of
high school, but forget that when it's your kid, right?" Daniel says
to me.

But it wasn't just that Jaxon was getting bad grades. The whole
family had been miserable and dysfunctional for a year. Now Jaxon's
issues had a name and a therapist was offering a solution. If stimulants
could fix Jaxon, Amy was game. More than game. Hadn't they tried
absolutely everything? She'd hung stuffed animals on her son! And
she did not want to risk Jaxon's getting booted from his school. His
crew of boys, including Collin and Kai, had been best friends since
pre-K. Leaving would also mean losing out on Chinese and severing
his link to his grandparents' homeland.

Education has always been a central tenet of the family's belief
system. Daniel was an activist for reform in the San Francisco public
schools while he was still a student in one. As a high schooler, he cam-
paigned against uniform periods of class length, believing that some
subjects demanded more time than others. At twenty-six, he ran for
the local school board. He lost. Now a venture capitalist, he's invested
over the years in companies that develop educational software. At one
point, years ago, he even tested a program designed for kids with
ADHD.

Amy's parents had emigrated from Hong Kong where they were
educated professionals. Her father was a mechanical engineer who
had worked for Levi Strauss and Co. Her mother was a high school
teacher. Her mother's parents were upper-class Chinese. Amy has a
picture of her grandmother as a little girl wearing gold chains around
her neck and waist.

Amy's mother was four when the Japanese invaded mainland
China during World War II. The family left their home, and, at one
point, while they were hiding in the mountains, Amy's mom remembers hearing a Japanese caravan move past on the road below them.

They eventually fled to Taiwan where they lived in crude military barracks provided by the government. Amy's grandfather, who'd studied accounting and economics at university, eventually rose to a job in the diplomatic corps. He spoke four languages, including Spanish, and was sent abroad to Peru.

When Amy's parents moved to San Francisco, before she was born, they slipped several rungs down the ladder. Limited by their poor English, they couldn't get jobs at the level equivalent to what they'd had. Amy's father was drawn to entrepreneurship, but his businesses never flourished. Amy's mother got work as a pre-K teacher's aide and supplemented her income by teaching cultural programs after school.

Amy grew up aware of how hard her parents worked. To their children they always seemed exhausted. Her dad traveled a lot. At one point he owned a Chinese food restaurant in Kansas while the family stayed behind in San Francisco. There were times when Amy's parents were holding down five jobs between the two of them, and yet, they could never work enough. They got by, but barely.

Like so many first-generation American kids, Amy understood that education was the only way she wouldn't end up struggling as her parents had. She'd have to pay for it herself. So at fourteen she started working after school and on weekends and during the summers. She was a clerk at a Chinatown souvenir shop and a stock girl for American Greetings, delivering cards to Bay Area drugstores. When she entered the University of California, Berkeley, she kept on working.

As she neared graduation, there was never a question that she'd continue with her education. She was driven less by a desire to pursue a certain career than by attaining financial security. She couldn't handle frog dissections in biology so medicine was out. She was already a business major, so getting an MBA seemed redundant. Law school it was.

In a single generation, Amy fulfilled her family's purpose, regaining for all of them their lost ground and then some. Before Jaxon was born, Amy and Daniel bought a 1920s Spanish-style home balanced high in the San Francisco hills, gutted it, then resuscitated it. Coated in a warm, buttermilk stucco, it's perched on the street like a bird on a lofty branch. Inside, their bookshelves are decorated with framed photographs of themselves next to smiling presidents, that rarefied design scheme available to political donors. When Jaxon was ten, he met President Obama, who asked how school was going. Jaxon's answer was: "Too much homework." The president was unsympathetic, saying, "Well, you've got to stick to it, buddy."

To Amy, the family still doesn't measure up. She speaks Mandarin, Cantonese, and English, and her children will know just Mandarin and English. "So we're not directionally correct," she says. It doesn't matter that many Americans don't know anything other than English. Compared to her grandparents' four languages, to Amy, her family is regressing.

Her education lifted her, but only so far. English was her third language, which meant she always had to work extra-hard. She was never able to get straight As. Once in her twenties she was talking to a law school friend of hers who used the word "epiphany." Amy had no idea what it meant. "That really brought home that there's an educational gap between someone like me who comes from an immigrant family versus someone who might have grown up with lawyers and judges as parents and grandparents. So I've always had a little bit of a chip on my shoulder about my English. I did growing up. Sometimes I still do," she says.

She started her law career as a prosecutor. Later, she was general counsel at a defense software firm that built simulation-training platforms for the Pentagon. Despite her professional success, the achievement she revels in (still!) is a high school test score: the four out of five she got on her AP history exam. "It was such a big deal to me because English wasn't my first language," she says. She makes fun of Daniel for getting a worse score on that same test even though he's fourth-generation American. "With all that you were given, you could only get a two," she says. Jaxon says his mom is always talking about that test.

Recently she had a slight career setback that brought on a wave of self-doubt. Her company merged with another one, and she was laid off. When she learned that the general counsel from the other company would be assuming her responsibilities, she looked him up online. "He went to better schools than I did. He was Phi Beta Kappa. He was top five percent of his law school class. He's got a ton more experience than I do. I happily defer to his, you know, greatness." She told her children, "I'm going to lose my job because I'm not as smart or as experienced as this guy, and I want you guys to remember that."

"That's not how you said it," Jaxon says. "You said, 'I'm losing my job because my brain's not valuable!'" Amy denies Jaxon's version, but she did seem to equate intelligence with grades and school reputation.

So by the time she, Daniel, and Jaxon walked into the pediatrician's office, Amy had one question for the doctor: "How soon can you put my kid on drugs?"

Dr. Sanford Newmark is tall and slim with a gentle voice and easy manner. A framed poster of Yosemite Valley and Half Dome's resplendent rock face joins the children's drawings taped onto his office wall. "One of my favorite places," he says not unwistfully. The UCSF professor of pediatrics, who told me leaky gut was real, specializes in ADHD as well as autism. At the UCSF Osher Center for Integrative Medicine, where he is the medical director of the clinic, he is also the head of the pediatric integrative neurodevelopmental program. In one of my first conversations with him, he marveled at the location of his practice, that a prestigious research institution like UCSF had embraced integrative medicine.

Amy had sent ahead forty-five pages of Jaxon's evaluations. At the appointment, Dr. Newmark spent about fifteen minutes chatting with Jaxon. How's school? Do you have friends? Then he dispatched him to the room next door to watch a movie.

Dr. Newmark turned to Amy and Daniel. "I would take Jaxon out of that school," he told them. "I would not recommend starting medication."

Wait. What?

"Your child might be borderline ADHD," Dr. Newmark said. "But you wouldn't be here if you went to another school."

"I didn't tell him I was on the board or anything," Daniel says now, chuckling.

Dr. Newmark suggested they read his book *ADHD Without Drugs: A Guide to the Natural Care of Children with ADHD*. At this, Amy groaned inwardly. She didn't need a doctor pushing a book on her. She thought, *He just wants my fifteen dollars*. Her second thought was, *You're going to make me do this before you give me the meds? That's fine. I'll do it because you'll give me the meds.*

At this point she and Daniel thought they'd exhausted all their other options. On the advice of a different doctor, Jaxon's longtime pediatrician, whom they'd seen the previous spring, they instituted regular walks and waited to see if Jaxon did better with a new teacher in the fall, among other strategies for dealing with ADHD. Nothing had made a major difference. When that doctor retired, the family sought out Dr. Newmark.

As Amy was thinking about the book she was going to have to buy, Dr. Newmark went on. "I see a lot of families from your school."

This got Amy's attention. Dr. Newmark told her he had fifteen to twenty students from their school in his practice, and he pointed out that he wasn't the only ADHD specialist in town. "So then that made it very scary," she tells me. It seemed to her like an outsized proportion. Amy suspected that the school was over-referring children for attention issues.

Dr. Newmark didn't think Jaxon's school was a good fit for him. "If kids have ADHD, academics tend to be hard," says Dr. Newmark, who spoke to me, with Amy's permission, late one afternoon in his office. "It's not their strength. Even if they're really smart. Just getting the work done and everything. So why put them in a place where they are going to be super-challenged? Why not just let them go to a sort of normal school?" His argument sounds astonishingly commonsensical.

"Think of what it's like for an ADHD kid at school," he says to me. "It's not fun. You're doing things that are hard for you all the time. It's like me. I'm a horrible artist. Imagine if I had to go to school all day, and I did art ninety percent of the time and reading ten percent. How would I feel about that? How would I feel about myself? Add to that tutoring and hours and hours of homework a night because they can't focus enough to get their homework done. You have to let them do things that are good for them, right?"

Our friend Dr. Rediger, the Harvard psychiatrist, who's not connected to Jaxon's case, tells me, "I think that sometimes we tend to look for a diagnosis when there's just a lot of stress in the kid's life. It's easier to diagnose the kid as being the problem and give him a medication than look at the problems with living that's really going on." Dr. Rediger says that there's some evidence that ADHD is connected to stress, but it's an understudied area.

Amy and Daniel had also wondered if the school wasn't part of the problem. They'd focused on its microscopic school yard, which they felt was inadequate for a boy who really needed to run around. And they had worried about the intense academic pressure. Starting in pre-K, students spend half the day learning in Mandarin. Then in fourth grade they switch from traditional Mandarin to a version of the language known as "simplified," a jarring shift that's like being transplanted from Shakespeare's England into modern-day America, Amy explains. It's a difficult transition for any child. As Jaxon's buddy Collin says about the language, "I mean I understand but I don't understand."

Daniel says that when he mentioned to the headmaster that he was thinking of pulling his children out of the school, the headmaster's response was, "You know, in the bigger scheme of things, your kid doesn't have to get an A in every subject. There's no such thing as the perfect student."

As comforting as it was to hear those words from the head of the school, it wasn't enough to defuse the culture of their community as Amy and Daniel experienced it. "It's a Chinese school, and the Chinese culture is very linear and single-minded," says Amy. "I'm totally overgeneralizing, but the culture of our school among the parent body is so incredibly uber–, ultra–tiger mom-ish," she says, referring to *The Battle Hymn of the Tiger Mother*, Amy Chua's bestselling book about being a demanding parent in the Chinese mold.

In fact, the pressure at Jaxon's school is so fierce that not even the Tiger Mother author herself could hack it there, Amy *Chan* says with a playful smile. "Amy Chua would get eaten alive at our school. Amy Chua is an amateur with no bragging rights," says Jaxon's mom. Not that she didn't inhale the other mother's book. Although she says she has consciously decided not to raise her kids à la Chua, she still questions whether she's doing them a disservice. "The headmaster can say we support all kids and we support all aspirations, but, at the end of the day, there is a bias against those who fall short in talent and commitment and aspiration," she says.

Amy and Daniel eventually abandoned the idea of switching schools. If they were torn about the intensity, the parts they loved about it— Jaxon's friendships, the language—won out.

Which is how they ended up in Dr. Newmark's office in the first place. They needed to make the school work for Jaxon.

AN ELIMINATION DIET AND THE GUT-BRAIN CONNECTION

Transferring Jaxon was just one suggestion. Dr. Newmark also wanted to try something that might directly tackle Jaxon's difficulty with focusing and controlling his impulses. He suggested an elimination diet.

For three weeks, Jaxon would stay off dairy, wheat, corn, soy, eggs, nuts, citrus, and any product with artificial colors, flavors, or preservatives. Then they would add the foods back in one by one and watch to see what happened.

Dr. Newmark believed that certain foods might be triggering Jaxon's ADHD symptoms. How it worked, he didn't know. But the connection between the gut and the brain is well established. Dr. Newmark explains that there are people with celiac disease, for example, who present with only neurological symptoms, such as fuzziness. Eating gluten is all it takes to set off a reaction. "There's a model in celiac disease and a huge amount of research about the idea that your gut is really your second brain," he says of the digestive tract, which is loaded with neurotransmitters, as well as neurons, that carry information up to the brain.

We've already discussed our gut, and how our bacteria are involved in so many aspects of our health. Scientists are starting to figure out how these resident microbes may influence how we act and feel, too.

Our gut bacteria population influences the body's level of the potent neurotransmitter serotonin, for example, which regulates feelings of happiness, as Justin and Erica Sonnenburg write in *The Good Gut*. "And serotonin is likely just one of numerous biochemical messengers dictating our mood and behavior that the microbiota impacts." Which itself is impacted directly, as we know, by what we eat.

Food sensitivities may be a factor. In 2006, researchers demonstrated that gluten sensitivity was a distinct medical condition—separate and unequal to celiac disease. Again it was Dr. Alessio Fasano's group, then located at the University of Maryland Medical Center, that made the discovery. If you have non-celiac gluten sensitivity and eat gluten, it can result in trouble throughout the body including diarrhea, bloating, cramping, abdominal pain, constipation, brain fog, depression, anemia, eczema, joint pain, osteoporosis, leg numbness, and ADHD-like behavior, Dr. Fasano writes in his book, *Gluten Freedom*. And that list is probably not complete, he tells me. Our understanding of non-celiac gluten sensitivity is where we were with celiac disease thirty years ago. "We know very few facts," Dr. Fasano says.

Dr. Newmark proposed experimenting with Jaxon's diet because there were no tests for diagnosing food sensitivities. In his own practice, he estimates that of the kids with ADHD who try the elimination diet, a third to a half significantly improve. He doubts the placebo effect is a factor. "If anything, a kid wouldn't want the elimination diet to work." He's not against prescribing medication to the kids who absolutely need it. He has some patients on medication who still stay off gluten, for example, because the wheat protein makes the problem worse.

"I think something about the gut's reaction to foods is producing either neurotransmitter changes or inflammatory markers. I think there's a big amount of communication between the gut and the brain and it produces substances that change brain function in some way. I'm not a neuroscientist. I just see what I see," says Dr. Newmark.

He's not the only one. Although the mechanism isn't understood, a number of studies testing elimination diets—some of which are stricter than what Dr. Newmark prescribes—have shown a positive effect in children with ADHD. In 2011, the authors of a randomized, controlled trial published in *The Lancet* concluded that the elimination diet had a "significant beneficial effect on ADHD symptoms" in 64 percent of the tested children. In 2012, a paper in *Pediatrics*, the main journal for pediatricians, surveyed the evidence—one of the cited studies found symptoms improved in 82 percent of the children; another one clocked in at 76 percent—and concluded, "In selected patients with diligent parents, a short 2- to 3-week period of restricted elimination diet is justified." There are the usual quality issues with these diet studies, though—small numbers, inability to rule out the placebo effect because you know what you're eating. So even if the risks are fewer, the evidence for diet is not as solid as what backs ADHD medications.

Dr. Newmark is baffled by the fact that the research on diet and ADHD isn't better known. "It's really kind of odd to me," he says. "I could go out and ask one hundred pediatricians right now whether diet works for ADHD and ninety-nine would say, 'No way. There's no research at all.'" How does he explain that? "Pharmaceutical companies," he says. I ask if perhaps well-meaning pediatricians just aren't keeping up with the latest research because it's practically impossible to. He agrees that there's an awful lot to wade through and that even though *The Lancet* is a top-notch journal, it's mostly geared toward adult medicine.

"But that's not the explanation," he says. "The explanation is that most doctors, I think, have a significant bias against nutrition. It starts in medical school. That's an important factor. It's taught horribly or not at all. Then when people get out into practice, the sad fact is that they get a great deal of their information from pharmaceutical reps. It's terrible, but it's true," says Dr. Newmark.

According to a *Pew Charitable Trusts Fact Sheet*, the pharmaceutical industry spent more than $24 billion on marketing to physicians in 2012, including the face-to-face meetings Dr. Newmark is referring to. The huge investment, though, doesn't mean doctors don't consult other sources. Dr. Aaron Kesselheim, a professor of medicine at Harvard Medical School who's written about the financial relationships between physicians and industry, says that while a large number of physicians do use drug reps as a resource, they also get information from continuing education and medical journals. Though continuing medical education (CME), which doctors need to maintain their licenses, is not untouched by industry money, either. "A good amount of it is sponsored by pharmaceutical and device companies," he says. "Although there are rules in place that are supposed to make sure that continuing education is independent, there's a worry that sponsored CME may have risks of bias."

Dr. Newmark goes on about his colleagues: "They also go to a lot of conferences, but many of these conferences are paid for by pharmaceutical companies," he says. Dr. Kesselheim says that sponsorship doesn't necessarily mean that drug companies have any say over what is presented at every single minute of the conference. "But it's an advertising tool," he says. "They are a presence."

Holly Campbell, the spokesperson for PhRMA, says, "Working together, biopharmaceutical companies and physicians can improve patient care, make better use of today's medicines, and foster the development of tomorrow's cures."

"Then there's the research," says Dr. Newmark. "Yes, those studies on diet and ADHD exist, but there's tons of research about medicines for ADHD. Most of it is short-term. But there it is. So it's a combination. I think people are well-meaning, but they start with a general bias toward pharmaceutical pills as opposed to nutrition and then you get that reinforced by drug reps. I think it's that combination that ends up with people not knowing about it, or if they hear about it, just dismissing it. Remember that the experts who put out the ADHD evidence-based guidelines are all people who make a lot of money from pharmaceutical companies. Or mostly, I don't want to say all. It's a horrible situation."

Is Dr. Newmark being unfair? I ask Dr. Mark Wolraich, a professor of pediatrics at the University of Oklahoma Health Sciences Center. He is one of the lead authors of the current American Academy of Pediatrics guidelines for treating ADHD as well as the recipient of payments, for speeches and consulting services, from four pharmaceutical companies that make ADHD medications, according to his own disclosures.

This makes Dr. Wolraich typical. A large majority of physicians—84 percent—have at least one type of financial relationship with a drug or medical device company, according to a survey published in 2010, conducted by Eric Campbell, a professor of medicine at Harvard Medical School who studies physician conflicts of interest. Dr. Campbell notes that the real figure is probably higher because people are likely to underreport something that's seen as inappropriate. "It's kind of like asking people how often they tell lies," he writes me in an email.

Dr. Wolraich says that the recommendation he made that children with ADHD—starting at age six—try medication and behavioral therapy first was based on the quality of the evidence for it. "I certainly agree with the criticism of most of the physicians in practice who may be getting their information from pharmaceutical reps." But Dr. Wolraich disputes the notion that he was paid "a lot" of money. Also: "I would take issue with the statement that those who participated in the guidelines are heavily influenced by pharmaceutical companies," he says.

Social science tells us that individuals tend not to be good judges of whether they're biased or not. Doctors are as susceptible to having this blind spot as are the rest of us, according to a 2003 *JAMA* commentary. "Bias is recognizable," the authors write, "but only in others."

DR. NEWMARK GREW UP IN New York City and started his career as a traditional pediatrician. But he'd always been interested in nutrition. He'd gone to college in the late '60s, early '70s. "There was the whole thing with, you know, back to the earth and alternative medicine," he says. He eventually did a fellowship at the University of Arizona Center for Integrative Medicine in Tucson.

But it was from a mom that he first learned the effect that diet could have on the brain. The year was 2000, when he was just beginning his fellowship. He'd had maybe two kids in his practice over the previous decade who'd had autism. He wasn't all that familiar with it. A mom came in with her four-year-old son who was flapping his hands and pacing back and forth. He didn't stop during the entire appointment. And he didn't speak.

The boy's mom said she wanted to try fish oil, probiotics, and a diet free of gluten and casein. "I thought, 'Why?'" says Dr. Newmark. "'What does diet have to do with autism?'" At the time the idea that taking certain foods out of autistic kids' diets might help their symptoms was out there, being talked about on support group message boards. Dr. Newmark just didn't know anything about it. The activist parents of autistic kids, by the way, are the godparents of all of us who've tried to find good answers for health problems on our own. Dr. Newmark went along with the mom's plan for her son, figuring it wasn't going to hurt the boy.

One month later the boy came back transformed. He still had autism, but he was dramatically better. He was making better eye contact, his hands were quiet, the chronic diarrhea he'd had his whole life had resolved. "I was like, 'Oh. There's something here,'" says Dr. Newmark.

THE THING IS, UNTIL THIS past century, diet was actually always a part of our medical regimen, going back to the writings of Hippocrates. If you showed up for a doctor's appointment in 530 BC in Athens or 1830 in Boston, a lot of the questions would have been relevant to various aspects of your lifestyle, including exercise and what you ate, says Dr. David Jones, who's a professor of the culture of medicine at Harvard Medical School. "These have been part of medicine for twenty-five hundred years. If you look at any medical textbook into the mid-nineteenth century, it's going to be full of information about diet as part of the therapy," he says.

I talked with him to get some context for Americans' tendency to look to pills to solve our health problems—doctors as well as their patients. He explained that while diet was an old therapeutic concept, so was the desire to find a pill that could cure everything. People were looking for a universal remedy in ancient Greece and medieval Europe. The idea gained steam again in the late nineteenth century, he says. A German researcher named Paul Ehrlich wrote to his colleagues that their goal as physicians was to find a magic bullet for bacterial diseases. It would address the disease and it would have no side effects.

When penicillin hit in the 1940s, it seemed to be the fulfillment of the prophecy, says Dr. Jones. For diseases like syphilis, antibiotics functioned just as Ehrlich had hoped, knocking it out with no negative consequences, at least none that we knew of then. "That's the precedent for all these other drugs."

The decade between 1945 and 1955 was a period of unmatched pharmaceutical discovery. The introduction of lithium as a mood stabilizer, diuretics for high blood pressure, modern chemotherapy for cancer, and many more antibiotics brought enormous confidence in the wonders of drug technology that we're very much living in the shadow of today. Fighting diseases with the right pill became the model. "The enthusiasm that follows from the decisive power of antibiotics has probably spilled over into other areas that it shouldn't," says Dr. Jones.

"We're neglecting all sorts of things that might help. If you get coronary artery disease, doctors know that you should lose weight and stop smoking. Many doctors do encourage this, but they are quick to prescribe statins and other drugs. If someone has obesity and diabetes, doctors will also encourage diet and exercise, but easily give up on this and move on to drugs and now bariatric surgery. These diseases are tied to nutrition, but doctors often have little faith in diet as part of a therapeutic regimen. Doctors now need to take diet more seriously as a central aspect of medicine, just as doctors have done for thousands of years," says Dr. Jones, who is a physician himself, a former practicing psychiatrist.

Why would intelligent professionals ignore evidence of an effective treatment, regardless of what it is? "There's a conspiracy theory that doctors are in cahoots with the pharmaceutical companies," says Dr. Jones. He believes that there may be some bad actors, but not enough to account fully for the general emphasis on prescribing something. The fact is: "It's easier to take a pill than to change a diet."

Another problem is that nutritional science doesn't have a lot of credibility. It's not nutrition's fault. Diet is hard to study, as Terry Wahls has discovered. There's also a pattern of reversals in the nutrition literature. Coconut oil was a bad oil. Now it's a good oil. A 2014 analysis of eighty studies involving more than a half million people contradicted long-held beliefs that the saturated fats found in meat, butter, and cheese led to heart attacks. The results, published in *Annals of Internal Medicine,* made headlines around the world. And then *that* study was called into question, with the nutrition chair at the Harvard School of Public Health suggesting it be retracted.

In the absence of overwhelming evidence, Dr. Newmark is the rare physician, who, like some of us laypeople, is comfortable experimenting with diet on an individual basis because it's not terribly risky. Why wait around for research that may or may not come?

AFTER AMY READ DR. NEWMARK'S book, she felt more open to trying out diet changes. In fact, the more she learned about ADHD, the more she wanted to put the brakes on medication. Dr. Newmark forwarded her a study of students in British Columbia concluding that the youngest boys in the class were 30 percent more likely to be diagnosed with ADHD than the oldest. For girls, the number was 70 percent. "So we're diagnosing immaturity," Dr. Newmark tells me.

Amy also learned from Dr. Newmark that the long-term effects of taking ADHD medications on a growing brain were completely unknown. "We're conducting a huge experiment on the brains of our children," he tells me. The known risks of popular stimulant ADHD medications include difficulty sleeping and loss of appetite. Some of the less common side effects are fainting, seizures, hallucinations, depression, slowed growth, and, rarely, sudden death. Ritalin, for example, is a federally controlled substance, classified as having a high potential for abuse and dependence.

There was maybe another factor, too, that made Amy comfortable with going against the norm. Like Terry Wahls and Jeffrey Rediger, she'd grown up on the outside of the mainstream and by now she was at ease there.

She'd been eager to medicate Jaxon because she thought it was the only option left. This new idea, that food could be a factor in her son's difficulties, rang true. Her parents had always been holistic about health. "That was part of my growing up. Foods have healing properties. In Asian cultures, there's always some herbal medicine that was a cure-all for blankedy-blank," she says.

Not that she bought into the supposed curative power of the various foods and herbal remedies her mother would push on her. "There is a specific herb that is believed to cleanse and dissolve blood clots," she says of Chinese herbal medicine. "And so it is believed that women should have this soup once a month right after their menstrual period. During high school and college, if I was around, my mom would automatically make it at the end of my cycle."

Amy would roll her eyes. "I didn't give it much credence," she says. And yet: "I'm very Americanized and Westernized, but in the back of my mind I believed in the connection between health and food."

Even so, neither she nor Daniel was convinced that changing Jaxon's diet would work because the data on it seemed thin. "But our view was: Why not try it?" says Daniel.

Still, they let Jaxon make the final call. Amy took a picture of the page in Dr. Newmark's book listing the eight foods they would be cutting out as part of the experiment. When she showed it to Jaxon on her smartphone, he was aghast. That year he'd been assigned to write a speech about something he loved. He had chosen eating as his topic. One paragraph was about how he loved eating bread. The next paragraph was about how he loved eating cake. The last paragraph was about how he loved eating candy—none of which he'd be enjoying, at least in their usual incarnations, on the elimination diet.

Amy and Daniel explained to him that medication would probably make it easier for him to study and do well in school. They also said that there was a possibility that it would change him completely, since it was a neurological drug and the long-term effects on developing brains weren't understood. They said that there was a very slim chance that he would stay exactly the same.

Jaxon didn't need any time to think about it. He looked at his parents. "I want to stay the same." He would not start medication.

"I was debating," Jaxon tells me. "But the real game changer was my mom saying, 'You won't be the same.' I didn't want to change my *mind*. I wanted to keep how fast my brain moves." It scared him to think about losing the things he liked about himself.

The psychologist counseled Daniel and Amy that it was unfair to ask a child to make medical decisions about himself, they say. "How is it not fair?" Jaxon asks when he hears this. "It's me!" He's furious at the idea that medication might have been imposed on him by adults. "They don't feel what you feel. You are the only person in the world that knows how you feel. Unless you're some psychic guy who has mind-reading skills with a machine that's like, 'Oh my God, I can feel how you feel and I can see your brain,'" he says. "There have been a lot of pointless things that adults have chosen that have been completely wrong."

We're sitting in the dining room. Occupying the center of the round table is a massive glass lazy Susan, like in a Chinese food restaurant. Just as we're talking about forbidden foods, Amy comes in with a bounty of everything Jaxon *can* eat. For dinner she's made gluten-free breaded pork chops, brussels sprouts, artichokes, and rice. Jaxon grabs a bottle of balsamic dressing as it whirls past him, pours some in a bowl, and says "I love my mom's artichokes" as he dips the spiky leaves in.

Eliminating certain foods is like saying goodbye to a loved one. "At first, I was in shock," says Jaxon. Then there was some irrational lashing out: "I hated Dr. Newmark," Jaxon says. Then bitterness showed up. "We had Thanksgiving lunch at school, which was the most wonderful time of my life!" And then, after enough time passes, there's the realization that it's not as bad as it used to be. "It only felt like that for eight months," Jaxon says of the hard times. And pretty soon he was in the arms of a new, if more stodgy, crush: an artichoke heart.

His family was well-positioned to make the transition to the new diet. At home, they already ate a largely non-Western menu. Amy tended to work with the vegetables, rice, and protein typical of Cantonese cuisine. In place of burners, half of her Viking range cooktop is occupied by a giant wok. She often roasted vegetables—kale, butternut squash, zucchini, cauliflower, or peppers—in seasoned salt and olive oil along with a rack of lamb or chicken. Tilapia was panfried and served over a bed of julienned ginger and green onions.

The launch of the diet still felt dramatic. Amy emptied her entire pantry and swept the shelves clean, just as Jamie Stelter had, then put back only qualifying food. She chucked her Pam spray oil because it contained wheat, soy, and artificial flavor. It was more difficult to part with other things, like her beloved Chinese shredded pork jerky, which had soy in it. "It took my mom three months to get rid of it," says Jaxon. "I still haven't gotten rid of it," she admits. It's in a jar hidden in the back of the fridge.

When the sandwiches Jaxon used to have for lunch became vegetables and rice left over from the night before, his friends noticed immediately. Growing boys that they were, this was a major development. Collin wanted to know what was going on. "I was like, 'What do you have for lunch?'" Collin tells me. "And he told me what he had. I'm just like, 'Normally you have different foods.' I'm just like, 'Why are you having this?' And he's like, 'Because I'm doing the elimination diet.' And I was like, 'Why are you taking a diet? You're so skinny.' He was like, 'It's not that kind of diet. It's because I'm ADHD.' I was like, 'What does that mean?' He explained, like, 'It means, like, I'm kind of, like, crazy? So I need to, like, eat these certain foods and supposedly it will help me, like, mellow down a bit.'" And, in the great tradition of uncomplicated boy relationships, that was basically it.

For a parent, taking eight foods out of a child's diet—there's really no other way to put this—is a huge pain in the ass. Amy might have been wary of medication, but it would have been a lot easier. But that's not the kind of reason that registers with her. "You should have seen her practice material for the bar," says Daniel. "Her notes were perfectly outlined. Her books had perfect tabs all color-coded, beginning to end. When she wants something, get out of her way."

The plan had been to try the diet for just three weeks, to see how it affected Jaxon's ADHD symptoms. If it didn't work, they'd turn to medication. Having a possible end date made an all-out effort feel more doable to Amy. "If I'm going to put him on medication for the rest of his life, I owe him my best effort for a three-week period! As a mom!"

ONE AFTERNOON NOT TOO LONG after starting the diet experiment, Amy picked Jaxon up from school and walked him across the street to one of their favorite cafés to do homework while Anderson was doing her after-school activities. Their latest routine was, once he got halfway through his homework, he could go order a big plate of French fries and a root beer, both okay on the elimination diet.

It was one of those early fall, Indian summer days San Francisco does so well. Amy and Jaxon were walking with their arms around each other. "He was asking about my day. He was telling me about his day. He was happy. He was being cuddly and sweet. He was not defensive or irritable. I remember thinking, 'Wow, he's such a great kid! This is really fantastic!' Both of us are really calm and happy to go to the café to do homework, and he was being polite and engaging and sweet and happy. It was such a huge deal. I don't know if it was a sunny day, but it felt like it was a beautiful, sunny day," Amy says. They were two weeks into the elimination diet, out of three. *Okay*, she thought. *Maybe there's something to this.*

At the same time Daniel noticed that the tension at home had cleared out. "The stress level in our house just went shooooo," he says, mimicking the sound of air fleeing a balloon. "He was completely like night and day. Before Amy would react and Jaxon would react and it would be like an echo chamber. So it would escalate. All that went away."

Jaxon's Chinese teacher noticed a change, too, and let Amy know. There were no noticeable shifts in his attention yet, but his energy was different, more steady, Amy says. In class, he had been buzzing around one second, crashing the next. On his previous Chinese test he'd gotten a 61. Two weeks into the diet, he retook it and got an 82. On the next test he climbed up to 92, then 98.

So when the three weeks were up and it was time to reintroduce one of the banned foods to see if it had any effect, Amy was hesitant. "I was a little bit afraid to let go of this. You know, the storm clouds had parted! The birds were singing! The sun was shining!"

Even so, she sent Jaxon to the store with his dad to pick out a loaf of bread, any one he wanted. Gluten was the first contestant. This being San Francisco, their local grocery store had an entire corner dedicated to sourdough, Jaxon's favorite. Jaxon plucked a round two-pound loaf the size of a restaurant dinner plate. At home, Amy unwrapped the spongy contraband. "It smelled really good," she says.

She cut it in half, then sliced a piece off from the big end. "He ate it, and he was super, super happy because he'd really missed it," she says. Amy and Daniel were sitting on either side of him at their dining-room table, watching. Jaxon kept chewing.

Just as he bit into his second slice, he started lifting his legs off his chair, like you do if it's a hot day and your thighs are sticking to the vinyl. It was as if Jaxon was trying to march while sitting down. "Daddy?" he said. "I'm not feeling good. I feel jumpy. I think I need to go for a walk." It was eight o'clock on a Saturday night. *"Now?"* Daniel said.

"I thought he was messing with us," says Amy. She and Daniel looked at each other. *Is this for real?*

Daniel and Jaxon headed out and came back three miles later. The next day they tried giving him sourdough again, and again Jaxon couldn't sit still. On his next Chinese test he got a 60. He grudgingly acknowledged that his favorite food seemed to be his kryptonite. Although, he points out, the effect gluten has on him is good for his soccer game. "Except for your concentration," says Daniel. "What?" says Jaxon. "Exactly," says Daniel. "You've got a lot of energy, but you're not looking at the ball."

*   *   *

JAXON WENT BACK OFF GLUTEN and moved on to testing dairy. (They had to try one food at a time to know its impact.) Daniel made lasagna with layers of mozzarella. Amy emailed Jaxon's teachers, as she'd done with the reintroduction of gluten, explaining where they were in the process and asking them to be on high alert. On Wednesday, one of his teachers emailed with an update. She reported that on Monday Jaxon had complained of being hungry and tired, as he'd done at the beginning of the year but not recently. On Tuesday he seemed sullen. He spent part of recess alone, which was unlike him. His ability to write independently, though, which had gotten better lately, still seemed to be fine. He needed reminders and frequent breaks but was less resistant than earlier in the year.

And then things got a lot worse. Another email arrived Wednesday afternoon. Jaxon was having trouble staying on task. Rather than work with his reading group, he went to chat with others or stand at the window. He didn't complete the assignment. After recess he said he couldn't concentrate and wrote only one phrase down in ten minutes. During math the students were supposed to be working independently. Jaxon stood up to get some paper, made a ball, and threw it across the classroom. When the teacher asked him to stop, Jaxon talked back. This was similar to how he'd acted at the beginning of the year, before the elimination diet experiment. That week he got a 54 on his test.

They kept going down the list, reintroducing various foods. Jaxon's scores and mood continued to zigzag. He was a terror on soy, reminding Amy of the Hulk, Mr. Hyde, *and* the Tasmanian Devil.

The forbidden foods seemed to make his life more difficult, but sticking to any diet, of course, is hard. One evening the family was out to dinner with Amy's sister's family and their parents at the Boudin Bakery in Fisherman's Wharf, which claims to be the birthplace of that dubious contribution to society, the bread bowl. Bakers push carts like gurneys full of the small, sourdough rounds from the ovens over to the prep counter to be disemboweled into vessels for chowder. Overhead, hooks continually moving along a system of tracks dangle baskets of additional loaves, like a dry-cleaning store for sourdough.

The tangy, yeasty aroma is irresistible, which is probably why the store puffs the warm, intoxicating vapors from its ovens out into the air through a vent positioned next to the sidewalk at the approximate height of a person's nose. Jaxon wasn't kidding when he talked about feeling taunted.

If this seems like an unkind choice of restaurant, Amy and Daniel didn't believe in shielding their children from challenges. Jaxon was a mature kid, and they gave him the responsibility they thought he could handle. This was why they wanted the diet to be Jaxon's decision. It was *his* health, after all.

Jaxon managed to order salad. Daniel left a good chunk of the bread bowl he'd gotten for himself on his plate. It was now soggy with soup. Jaxon gazed at it. The bread gazed back. "My mom's like, 'You can't eat it. You can't eat it. You can't eat it,'" says Jaxon. "I was depressed." Then Amy and Daniel stepped away from the table. They consulted privately, and then they came back and said, "If you can really control yourself, then we'll let you have one of our bread bowls." Jaxon tells me, "I just jaw-dropped." He did eat it, and it made him feel sick.

Once the experiment was over, they concluded that Jaxon had a problem with six out of the eight forbidden foods. (Corn and citrus didn't seem to bother him.) Their impressions were that the individual foods had very distinct effects on him. Gluten: "I just bounce around and I can't concentrate." Dairy: "Dairy makes me irritable." Soy: "What it looks like for me is *rrroooaaarrr.*"

Remember how Daniel said the stress level in their house bottomed out? It turned out that Jaxon didn't do it all on his own. Amy had also gone off dairy, wheat, soy, eggs, nuts, corn, citrus, and artificial additives. It was how the whole family ate at home. She came to believe that nuts, particularly, had contributed to her anger. "She goes on rampages," says Jaxon. "I can tell you all about it. She acts so explosive."

Amy had also suffered from nasal allergies her whole life. "Immediately before starting the elimination diet I was on four daily allergy medications for my sinuses, having no relief. I was on Flonase. I was on Mucinex. I was on Sudafed. And I was on ibuprofen. I was on so much Sudafed that I'm sure I'm on somebody's list," she says, because an ingredient in Sudafed is used in making methamphetamine. She hasn't taken anything since she went on Jaxon's diet. She also used to have regular outbreaks of eczema on her hands. It cracked open the skin on her knuckles, "like a capital I," right along the joint. Now all of that is gone.

Anderson had always had eczema, too. Amy started eyeing what her daughter was eating for possible triggers. A particularly awful flare-up after gluten-free, dairy-free pancakes—"My knees were plump, cherry, delicious red," Anderson says—led to a suspicion of the coconut yogurt used in the batter. Cutting it out did the trick. That left Daniel. Nothing much to report, but he does feel less bloated! "Gluten makes me a little more sleepy in the afternoon," he says.

Dr. Newmark hears about the collateral benefits of the diet all the time from families. "I saw this girl. I can't remember what she came in for, but she had some eczema. But her mom had the worst eczema you could imagine. Her hands looked like slabs of raw meat. She'd been to every dermatologist, had every treatment imaginable. So I put the kid on this gluten-free, casein-free diet. She comes back in a couple months. The kid's better but Mom's hands were cured. This one was amazing. She was so happy." He hears about all sorts of issues clearing up: constipation, diarrhea, GI upset, IBS symptoms, fuzziness, fatigue, and bloating. Bloating is a big one. "I never knew bloating was such a problem!" he says. It can be caused by a number of things, including gluten intolerance. Certainly the placebo effect could explain some of the resolution. "But not all," says Dr. Newmark.

Even once they'd figured out which foods seemed to bother Jaxon, all of his issues weren't solved. For one thing, compliance, especially at the beginning, is more difficult than you'd think. One week while Amy was out of town for work, she got an email from Jaxon's English teacher. Jaxon is having a hard time focusing in class, she said, and is not getting any work done this week. He is continually getting up and disturbing others. Is there anything different going on? Amy checked in with Daniel. He insisted he was executing the diet perfectly.

When Amy got home, she found a "ginormous" bottle of vegetable oil in the cupboard. She was furious. It contained soybean oil. "This is vegetable oil!" Daniel said, a guilty man still professing his innocence. "You actually have to read the ingredients list," Amy said. "That's what being on this diet is."

As fourth grade progressed, it remained a rocky year for Jaxon. Home life was tranquil. The diet seemed to have brought back a nicer kid. But the diet changes didn't instantly turn Jaxon into a perfect student. Food isn't a magic bullet, either, of course. Fourth grade was, after all, the year that students had to transition to simplified Mandarin, which made it a lot harder than other years. Amy was seeing promise, but his grades weren't consistently good.

That spring, Amy started wondering about medication again. *If this was the most the elimination diet could do for him, maybe it wasn't going to be enough,* she thought. "It breaks my heart to see the range in his grades," she told me at the time. "When I see the 80s and 90s, I see the potential. Intellectually I tell myself I don't want to medicate him to see the 90s. But I still struggle emotionally. I think, 'If I medicated him a little bit, can I get him into Harvard?' It's not that I want my child to go to Harvard. I want my child to have the choice to go to Harvard."

As the year went along, they experimented with other tools to help Jaxon in the classroom. Jaxon tried using an iPad for writing assignments, which resulted in a multifold increase in his output. He sat on a balance ball in class, which was also effective, until he and his friends popped it while horsing around. He sat in the library away from everyone. He got a Chinese tutor. All of this helped.

These strategies coincided with a major shift in perspective at the school. "Historically the school wasn't very tolerant of kids with different needs," says Daniel. The head of school, who was new, felt that it had to be more adaptive to individual learners rather than the other way around, says Daniel. So they brought in specialists to work with teachers on how to deal with different sets of kids. Letting Jaxon use an iPad for writing instead of being sent to the counseling office and told to get in line was part of that. The family came to believe that the diet was a major contributing factor to Jaxon's success at school, but it wasn't everything.

Still, everyone who knew Jaxon well noticed a difference in him. Amy says that the music teacher pulled her aside and said, "I'm really glad you did this." His science teacher saw a huge improvement. Hearing that from someone who'd taught him three years in a row was especially gratifying for Amy.

Jaxon's friends are also appreciative. "He doesn't get as angry anymore," says Kai. "He's not as hyper," Collin says. "Since he's been doing the elimination diet I think he's been focusing better." Jaxon still talks a lot—the two sit next to each other in class—but Collin devised a system to deal with it. He keeps a table football on hand, a triangle made of folded Post-it notes and tape. If Collin is trying to pay attention to the teacher and Jaxon wants to tell him that he found fifty diamonds playing Minecraft the night before, Collin just flicks the football at him.

Jaxon used to be the one who got pulled out of class. Now he watches while other kids get yanked. I ask him how that feels and he exhales. "I'm not the only one!" he says. He says that it felt "so good" to get good grades and that he was proud of himself. He punches the air. "These are 'yay!' punches," he says.

One thing to consider: If immaturity can be misconstrued as ADHD, it's certainly possible that things got smoother for Jaxon simply because he grew up.

Amy feels enormously grateful for Dr. Newmark. She's not a particularly religious person, but she feels there may have been some greater being or force, something she doesn't understand, that connected her family to him.

But, of course, he didn't help Jaxon on his own. Amy and Daniel had to be willing partners. "I can choose to work hard and expend my energy in pursuit of whatever leads, however promising, or I can choose not to. And I choose to expend my energy that way for my child. Because no one else is going to. You have to be your child's best advocate, your child's crusader. Doctors have a lot of patients to take care of, and they can't be single-minded. Maybe it's a snobbery that we single-handedly can make a difference," she says. "A snobbery believing that we're the only one in the current situation who have the power and the brains and the brawn to make a difference."

WHEN JAXON ENTERED SEVENTH GRADE, his behavior and attitude at home remained "phenomenal," Amy says. His teachers still reported some disruptive behavior in class—talking out of turn, swiveling in a swivel chair, if that counts—but his grades continued to be in the 80s and 90s.

That same year, three years after his initial diagnosis with ADHD, Jaxon was due for a follow-up assessment. Amy was curious if the educational psychologist's measurements would reflect the changes in Jaxon they all had noticed.

The retest looked at the same range of factors including cognition, memory, focus, and executive function. Though his grades had improved at school since before he started the diet, the results of the psychologist's tests did not show a change in the areas of weakness identified before. Jaxon's strengths, however, had grown even more muscle. His verbal skills, for example, now tested at a college level. How to explain the positive change in Jaxon's academic performance when his scores on factors related to ADHD hadn't gotten better? Perhaps his improvements in other areas balanced the overall picture. Pediatricians say that the brighter children are, the better they're able to compensate. And these tests may not be accurately measuring the factors that most strongly affect school and life performance in those children with ADHD.

Still, Amy was disheartened and "briefly, very, very briefly" toyed with the idea of ditching the diet. When she talked it over with Jaxon, though, the two of them agreed that their own assessment—that he simply felt better on a daily basis—was not to be discounted, even if it wasn't picked up by the psychologist.

In Amy and Daniel's conversation with the psychologist about the results, he asked if they wanted to consider medication, they say. When Amy and Daniel took Jaxon in for an appointment, Amy mentioned the idea of medication. Jaxon broke down. "Mom, you said you were happy with my As and one B in Chinese. Why are you now pushing to medicate me? I have to work really hard to get that B. I have to give everything. Please let that be okay," he said. "I don't want to be medicated. Why can't I be who I am?"

Amy was immediately persuaded by her son's words and started crying. She says the educational psychologist also teared up. Amy tells me that it's Jaxon's decision whether to be medicated or not and that she supports his choice not to be.

Maybe this was the person Jaxon was always going to be, or maybe he was shaped by the efforts of the previous three years—bucking the standard of medicating ADHD children, choosing the harder, untraveled path. Either way, it was certainly evident in the psychologist's office who he was now, a twelve-year-old boy with a strong sense of himself and quite a lot of fight.

Jaxon has started touring high schools even though it's ahead of schedule. He has a clear vision of a small school with diverse teachers and kids who appreciate and celebrate each other's uniqueness—kids who want to stay the same.

13

Amy Thieringer

Evolution of a Healer

That thought, that I might not be successful, never entered my head.
That's not the way I think. The way I think is, "Okay. What do I
want to do?"
—AMY THIERINGER

AMY THIERINGER, WHO STEPPED PAST THE LIMITS OF MEDICINE TO take on Amanda Hanson's son's allergies, wasn't an obvious candidate for savior. She had no medical training. In school, she wasn't even good at science. But like others in this book, she was forcefully independent and had gumption to spare, so unlikelihood didn't interfere with her purpose. As she developed Allergy Release Technique, her unique background and outsider status would even turn out to be an advantage.

Amy wasn't born a rebel. As a little girl she stuck close to what was expected of her. She was shy and unsure of herself, and the confines that rules provided were comforting; she had no inclination to loosen their embrace. "I wasn't pretty. I was awkward," she tells me. And her mother let her know. She used to say to Amy, "Ugly in the cradle means pretty at the table!," meaning that Amy would grow into her features. This was supposed to be encouraging.

She grew up in an expansive home on the golf course in Brockton, Massachusetts, outside of Boston. The walls were made of sliding glass doors. Her parents had spent several years building it.

They filled their new house with screaming and yelling. The mood in the home was always tense. "Very sparky," Amy says. The clashes weren't about anything specific. "It was everything, you know," Amy says. Witnessing these conflagrations, Amy and her two brothers were inevitably singed. And sometimes, Amy remembers, verbal abuse came right at them.

"We were fighting, but there was also a lot of love and support for Amy as she developed into who she is today," says Amy's mother. "Some of the fighting and the tension was because we were getting a divorce and we almost lost our youngest son in a bike accident." Amy's father did not respond to requests for comment.

As a teenager, Amy started sneaking out at night while everyone was asleep—sliding glass doors make their own *sh* sound. A whole group of kids would be waiting at the end of the street, spring-loaded for carousing.

Amy's friends were disaffected rich kids, and she emerged as a leader. They skipped class and went roof-riding—someone drove, someone rode belly-down on top of the car, with only the rack to hold on to. They got drunk and smoked pot. Amy wore Sasson jeans that were so tight she had to lie down on her bed to zip them up. She layered pastel button-downs—pink on yellow on white—like a petit four. Like Amy, eighties fashion was just getting going.

Amy's family had money. Her grandfather, Max Coffman, was a discount-department-store tycoon. The son of Russian immigrants, he'd gotten his start as a grocery store delivery boy. According to his *Boston Globe* obituary, he boxed on the streets for extra money, collecting nickels from passersby.

In the 1950s, he went into business for himself, opening the first store that would grow into the Mammoth Mart chain. His innovation was to put the cash registers at the front of the store, like he'd seen at the Stop & Shop market where he used to work. At the time, most department stores had you pay for your shoes in the shoe department and your gloves in the glove department. Coffman got rid of all those counters and salespeople and promoted the cost-saving idea of self-service. Meanwhile he hooked his cash registers up to computers that tracked what was selling and what wasn't.

As Mammoth Mart was taking off, a young Sam Walton was getting started on his own brand of no-frills store. He'd opened only three of them when he sought out the advice of Coffman, according to the *Globe*. Coffman's son, Jeffrey, gave Walton a tour of a store. The Mammoth Mart chain eventually grew to nearly ninety stores up and down the East Coast.

Amy was not close to her grandfather, but the lessons of his success were in circulation while she was growing up: The fact that he'd done well despite not having graduated from college. That he'd been an outsider with a good idea. That he'd made it all happen through hard work. "He was a really smart guy," she says. "In a really different way. He was an innovator. I knew that about him."

By the time Amy was a junior in high school, she was in the thick of her rebellion. She'd never excelled in academics, but now her grades were getting worse. She was seeing a therapist then, and the work helped her realize where she was headed. She came to understand that the path of sneaking out, drinking, and doing drugs, which she'd taken to get away from unhappiness, would eventually lead her right back to its door.

She needed to quit her social scene and find a more effective escape from her home life, a more permanent one. She needed, she thought, to go to boarding school.

Her parents refused to send her.

Amy refused their refusal.

For years, the troubled family had gone to group counseling sessions at a therapist's home. At one meeting, attended by her family and others, she read aloud a letter she'd written outlining why she needed to get out of her house. "The only way I can be okay is to go to boarding school. And I know you can afford it," she said.

The room exploded in applause—only Amy's parents weren't clapping. The therapist announced, "She's going!" Amy's mother says that she and Amy's father came to agree that it was worth trying. That fall, Amy left home and enrolled in Wykeham Rise School for Girls in Washington, Connecticut. She gave up the partying and became an A student. "It was my first experience of myself as smart," she says.

IT TURNED OUT THAT AMY was fleeing not only her dysfunctional family but her own early history. When she was nine years old, she says she was sexually assaulted by a trusted person in her life who is now deceased. As with many people who experience childhood trauma, Amy buried the memory and kept it hidden even from herself. That didn't take care of the misery, though, which drifted to the surface. It wasn't until Amy was in her late thirties that intensive therapy unearthed the full extent of what had been troubling her.

The revelation of what she'd gone through as a child undid her. Sometimes she wondered if what she thought had happened to her had actually happened. "You question it because it's something you completely disassociated from and suddenly it feels real, like, really real."

The notion of repressed memories is controversial. According to the American Psychological Association, most leaders in the field believe that a memory of early trauma can be remembered later after having been forgotten, though it is a rare occurrence. Experts agree that it is also possible to construct convincing false memories. Amy says she ultimately experienced healing as a result of grappling with her memories.

Once the earlier trauma surfaced, she kept reexperiencing it. She felt like she was underwater and couldn't reach the surface to get air. It was like being waterboarded by her past.

She was diagnosed with post-traumatic stress disorder and saw several therapists before finding the right one. The first therapists, Amy says, would take the cap off too quickly. All the bad stuff would shoot out. "Everything [was] just rushing and that's why you get all the panic," she says. Once she was in the care of another therapist, she learned that traumatic events had to be tiptoed up to, very carefully, very lightly, a lesson she'd take with her into her work.

BEFORE AMY BECAME INTERESTED IN curing allergies, she was interested in fashion. During college she interned for the merchandising department of Talbots, the women's apparel company. She was later hired after graduating from college, eventually becoming a buyer and catalog stylist. When she arrived, the company was just transitioning to computers. Amy taught her colleagues how to use them. Then she wrote an algorithm that would allow the merchandisers to keep track of how much cash they had on hand each month, to know how much more merchandise they could afford to buy. It was similar to what her grandfather had instituted in his stores, though she says she wasn't aware of it at the time.

When she was twenty-six, she married a nice man in the Domino's Pizza franchise business. She'd always wanted to be a mom, and they had three children together. "He was a pretty laid-back, Midwestern guy," she says. Amy was more expressive and emotional and the clash of their personalities—and no doubt the invisible baggage she was lugging around—weighed down the marriage and eventually crashed it. Once issues between them arose, Amy wanted to deal with them, she says. "He wanted out pretty quickly." Their children were three, five, and seven.

After her divorce, she was set up on a date with a naturopathic physician and complementary medicine practitioner. It was her first introduction to unconventional ideas about healing. A therapy workshop he recommended to her had a very holistic perspective, and she readily embraced it. "It was very much about connecting to your soul, connecting to the universe," she tells me. The two would eventually marry.

In my conversations with Amy, which took place over three years, I found that I often needed something she said to be translated. At one point she was talking about what she learned in therapy. "Through that I connected to myself," she said. I asked her, "Can you explain that more?" Her answer, accompanied by a laugh, was: "No." Then she gave it a try. "It was the opening of my life to connect to myself, my spirit to be able to listen to my intuition."

And then she says: "Where you want to see your life going."

It was at a naturopath conference that she went to with her second husband that Amy first met the little machine that she would later use in her practice. It was marketed as a tool that used acupuncture points to see what was out of balance in the body. Amy didn't find it the least bit baffling when she first encountered it. "Why don't you get one?" Amy asked her husband.

He ended up buying a BioScan device, as it is now called, for his practice. (The price tag today is upward of $12,000.) Amy got training and started working with her husband, using the machine to do evaluations of clients. It turned out that the woman who wrote algorithms for the Talbots merchandising department was a natural with this electronic equipment, too. Her husband, the naturopath, would then prescribe various supplements to the patients.

Amy is well aware of how talking about unbalanced energy can sound to certain audiences. Years ago, when the Boston-based chef Ming Tsai was quoted in the press talking about taking his son to an energy healer named Amy Thieringer, she called him up. "You can't call me that in public," she told him. "It will make people think I'm a nut."

Amy wasn't concerned about whether or not there was evidence for what she was doing. When she unburied the trauma in her past, she realized that, before, her entire understanding of her personal history had been wrong. Facing the truth of what she had gone through as a child taught Amy to question the dominant narrative. What she trusted most now was herself.

So when Amy heard that there was a new protocol a chiropractor had developed that promised to get rid of severe allergies, she was open to it and interested in learning how to do it. Only months before, she'd sped to the ER with her thirteen-year-old son after he'd eaten three cashews and started having trouble breathing. He'd never had an allergic reaction before. At the hospital he was given a shot of epi-nephrine and was discharged with strict instructions never to have tree nuts again. She was told that there was nothing else that could be done to protect her son.

At least, that was the dominant narrative.

The new therapy was called NeuroModulation Technique, or NMT. It purported to be a mind-body treatment for a number of problems, in addition to allergies, that Amy would later incorporate into her own approach. In NMT, the idea is to get the mind to recognize the mistake the body is making by attacking an innocent food as if it were an invader.

Scientists use the term "neuromodulation" to mean changing how brain cells operate—the speed at which they fire. The most direct way to affect a neuron is to zap it with electricity, as in electroshock therapy. The most familiar method probably is drugs—Prozac, Ritalin, and others—which also regulate the firing of brain cells, often by binding to them. And as the University of Colorado's Steven Maier told us, talk therapies can change the brain, too; that's why they work for anxiety and depression.

NMT—the therapy—doesn't come from science. To me, it sounds like ESP. Here's how its creator, Leslie Feinberg, described it to me in an email: "In NMT, we directly communicate with the mind-body directly [sic], using intention rather than speech as we would in a conscious level dialog." The website has an "As Seen on TV" vibe: "Introducing the all new NMT PainEraser!"

With Amy's new open sensibility, the mechanics of NMT did not give her any pause. It was around 2005 when she flew to Florida for a three-day training session in the practice. She'd experienced the horror of an anaphylactic allergic response firsthand. She wanted to be able to help children like her son.

Also, she and her second husband were on the outs. She knew she was going to need to set up her own practice.

Did it occur to her that she wasn't the most likely candidate to help kids overcome severe allergies, the promises of NMT training aside? "That thought, that I might not be successful, never entered my head. That's not the way I think. The way I think is, 'Okay. What do I want to do?'"

One of her first clients was the chef Ming Tsai's son, David, an almost five-year-old who had multiple food allergies. David's mom, Polly, had first taken him to see Amy's husband, the naturopath. Polly remembers that the naturopath prescribed a lot of supplements, which was a lead-up to trying to reintroduce certain foods David was allergic to. Eventually, according to Polly, the naturopath placed a piece of matzo on David's lip. Though he'd recently tested negative for wheat, tests can be inaccurate, and David immediately broke out in hives.

According to Polly, the naturopath quickly ushered David into another part of the office where Amy was working and asked her, "Can you do something?" (The naturopath does not recall the incident.)

Amy used her new NMT training to try to convince David's body that wheat was nothing to be afraid of. She whispered a message to his brain, tapped him on the back, had him breathe in and out; the hives faded away. Sometimes hives last for only minutes, but Polly was impressed.

Amy told Polly that the next time they'd give the matzo another go. Polly was thinking, "No way it will work," but she did go back. "I was grasping at straws at that point." Here was another mom shoved into trying new ways to help her child, in desperation.

Polly wanted to do everything possible that she thought was safe. Her father was a physician, and she had worked as an RN. She had always been very open-minded about therapies and interested in Eastern medicine. Before she met Amy, she'd taken David to various practitioners including an acupuncturist and someone trained in NAET (Nambudripad's Allergy Elimination Techniques), just as Amanda Hanson had.

When Polly took David back to see Amy the following day, she stood over her son double-fisting—Benadryl in one hand, an EpiPen in the other. Though what she said was indecipherable to any listener, Amy told David's brain that his body needed to stand down, that this was just wheat, and it wasn't going to hurt him. She put the cracker on David's lip again and this time there was no reaction at all. Polly looked at her. All she said was, "Amy."

Amy was blown away, too. "It was the first time that I'd seen what I did actually work," she says. "It was a big uh-huh, a big wow."

Although children often outgrow their allergies to wheat, for it to have happened to David right on cue seems unlikely. It's impossible to know what it was that kept him from having a physical reaction. Was it the NMT? Or was it Amy's absolute confidence that she could do it, that key ingredient of the placebo effect?

When Amy left both her marriage to the naturopath and his practice, she took with her only three things: the BioScan machine and contact information for two clients, one of whom was Polly.

Polly and her son went to see Amy every week at her new office in her home and, later, in space rented from a physical therapist. They started with the foods that David had never had a severe reaction to. They worked their way down the long list, which included soy, eggs, and peanuts. David learned to tolerate all of them without a problem.

Dairy would be the real test since David had once had an anaphylactic reaction to it. It had happened less than a year earlier. He was at his grandfather's eightieth birthday party. A babysitter gave him milk, and his throat started to close. It would also be the first time Amy would try introducing a food that had been so dangerous.

Amy dipped a toothpick into ice cream and smeared a tiny drop of it onto David's lip. His response was immediate. "It's tingling! It's burning!" he said. He panicked.

He'd been pretty calm when Amy had reintroduced the other foods. He'd never gotten upset like this before. And yet, his behavior was familiar to Amy. The fear. It was as if David was at that birthday party again, reliving that earlier trauma when his throat threatened to choke off his breath, a needle was jabbed into his leg, and his parents hovered over him, frantic.

That was it. Looking at this little boy, his heart beating so fast, Amy saw herself. The ice cream had triggered more than a memory in David, she believed. He seemed to have been dragged back into a terrified state, just as she had experienced after realizing she'd been assaulted. David could have died the last time he was exposed to dairy. Amy was sure that he had PTSD stemming from that earlier event and was now being subjected to a flashback or severe anxiety as a result.

David eventually calmed down. His lip felt normal again, and he did not need medical attention. But before resuming the therapy, Amy decided to do some more research.

She called a psychotherapist she knew who specialized in trauma. She wanted to learn more about how the brain worked. She arranged to pay the therapist for consultations. She wanted to explore whether David's anxiety related to dairy could trigger the physical tingling he felt, and, more to the point, *if she could treat the anxiety, would that help the allergy go away?*

After a couple of meetings with that first therapist, Amy met Leslie Brody, the director of the Emotion, Gender, Culture & Health Laboratory in the Department of Psychological and Brain Sciences at Boston University. She was also a clinical psychologist who treated children and adults with anxiety and mood disorders, some of whom also had allergies.

Anxiety often accompanies allergies, which makes sense because our fight-or-flight response evolved to protect us from danger. If you spot a crocodile at the watering hole, you'd be advised by your trusty nervous system to clear out before you even have to think about it. In the same way, if you've learned that a food can kill you, you're preprogrammed to run for your life—or at least get shot through with the adrenaline rush that could fuel your sprint.

In her lab at BU, Brody has focused her research on how psychological and physiological processes interact and affect each other. She and her colleagues have looked at the effect of psychosocial factors on immune function, specifically in women with HIV who participated in the federally funded Women's Interagency HIV Study covering a twenty-year period. Her work suggests that the amount of HIV in the bloodstream of infected women is related to their emotions and behaviors. In one study she found that women who were hiding their infection carried a higher viral load, which has also been shown to be true of men who were hiding both their HIV and the fact that they were having sex with other men. Depression also correlated to higher levels of HIV. All of it suggested that the mind could influence our bodily processes—and vice versa.

Leslie Brody had come to Amy for help with her own allergies. She'd developed a number of food and environmental allergies as an adult. The only treatment that traditional Western medicine had offered her was avoidance. But some of her main triggers—pollens, dust, and mold—were everywhere.

Brody heard about Amy from an acupuncturist who knew of Amy's work through other clients. As a scientist, Brody was naturally hesitant about working with someone whose procedures were as untested as Amy's were. Brody tells me in an email, "Her treatment was not empirically evaluated and was not particularly understandable within existing scientific theoretical frameworks." She adds, "Even less so than acupuncture!"

Brody was reluctant to invest time and money in something that might not work. But her life was becoming hemmed in by her worsening allergies. She could eat only a few foods without having digestive or respiratory symptoms and had lost more than thirty pounds. She might as well find out more about what Amy did.

Amy gave Brody the names and numbers of two adults she'd worked with who had similar environmental allergies. One of the women told Brody that Amy's treatments had been lifesaving for her and that she had found the machine Amy used to be very accurate in identifying triggers for her allergic symptoms.

Amy herself inspired confidence over the phone, Brody says. She got the sense that Amy would listen and that it would be a collaborative process.

Over several months, Amy used her BioScan machine to test three hundred different foods and environmental substances without knowing Brody's ideas about what affected her. Out of that number Amy pinpointed the ten that Brody knew to give her the biggest problems as well as the few foods that she could actually eat without becoming reactive, including—incredibly—something as specific as Havarti green beans.

Brody was amazed by the results. She told Amy, "I'm beginning to trust your machine." Amy retorted, "Well, I'm beginning to trust that you're accurate in knowing what you're allergic to."

It would take five years to work through Brody's long list of allergens, but in the end, she was able to tolerate almost everything with occasional tune-ups needed in the form of electrical stimulation to acupuncture points. She adds, though, that she thinks it was not Amy's treatment alone that made a difference. She was doing many other things that she believes helped, including eating fermented foods and doing traditional acupuncture.

It's tempting to speculate that Brody might have gotten better without treatment in those five years—with time alone doing its healing work—but she thinks it's unlikely given that she had been sick for at least as many years before consulting Amy, and people with similar health conditions report them as being chronic.

Amy benefited from the relationship, too. She had the raw intelligence and the insight, but Brody was her link to the science of how the body worked. Amy's inkling about David Tsai, that his physiological reaction to the ice cream was triggered by fear alone, dovetailed with her new client's research at the Emotion, Gender, Culture & Health Lab at BU.

Amy dropped the first consultant she'd sought out and started collaborating with Leslie Brody soon after they met.

When Amy wasn't working on Brody's sensitivities, the two met sometimes twice a week to discuss how Amy might be able to treat allergies by tackling what she viewed as the PTSD component. Amy already knew that the previous trauma had to be approached slowly and deliberately. Rush into it and panic could erupt, just as she'd experienced and just as she'd seen in David Tsai.

Given her research about the relationship between psychological and physiological processes, trying to address the panic and anxiety involved in an allergic reaction made sense to Brody. She had had a lot of success using cognitive behavioral therapy in her own practice, teaching her patients to step back and notice anxious thoughts as they arose as a guard against getting carried away by a storm of panic. A lot of us know this practice by its other name: mindfulness. Another important part of CBT is to be cognizant that the anxious reaction will pass. According to the VA's National Center for PTSD, cognitive behavioral therapy is the most effective type of counseling for PTSD specifically.

Brody adapted the practice for Amy, to make it specific to allergies. "Amy was always open to improving upon the treatment to help as many people as possible," Brody says.

So with Brody's guidance Amy started teaching the children she was working with to recognize what an anxious reaction looked and felt like. She told them that anxiety was the body's protective defense against substances it registered as dangerous. Borrowing from the practice of mindfulness as well as from Internal Family Systems therapy—a treatment for trauma that focuses on connecting with multiple parts of the self—Amy taught the children first to thank the protective/anxious part of themselves. Then they were instructed to let that part know that they appreciated what it was trying to do but not to work so hard. These were the firefighters that Amanda Hanson's son, Hayden, had learned to call off.

The kids were also encouraged to come up with positive coping statements or mantras such as "I am safe," "I don't have to protect myself," or "This food is delicious and I want to enjoy it." Amy asked them to identify times when they had felt strong and brave and, at those moments when the anxious part made an appearance, to remember those better times. Because tapping acupressure points could have a calming effect, it was to be done at the same time as the kids were focusing on the memory, to underscore the idea of safety.

Amy reminded the children she worked with that they could cope with allergic reactions if and when they happened by tapping, taking Alka-Seltzer Gold or Benadryl, or using an EpiPen.

Brody had learned about the effectiveness of alkaline substances, such as Alka-Seltzer Gold, in calming down inflammatory (allergic) processes from fellow allergy sufferers and a doctor in Boston who specialized in immune dysfunction and environmental illnesses.

The addition of cognitive behavioral therapy ideas to Amy's protocol was critical. It allowed her potentially to decrease a child's autonomic nervous system arousal, which drives the fight-or-flight response, and empower him or her to tolerate or regulate the anxiety that often accompanied and exacerbated the allergic process. The result was that the reintroduction of allergens started to be a much smoother, faster process.

After David Tsai had panicked, Amy had taken a break from trying to reintroduce dairy to him. Once she figured out how to use CBT, she pulled her pint of ice cream out again. This time, it worked.

It took David five years to graduate from Amy's care. When he turned sixteen, he entered his seventh year of being able to eat anything. But kids, like Hayden Hanson, who started the process later—after Amy had developed her protocol more fully—now can get through a lot faster.

One of the first allergic children to try out the revised protocol was Jacob Epstein. At nine months old, Jacob was given formula for the first time. He sucked it down and passed out. Skin tests at the hospital suggested extensive allergies. The doctor told Jacob's mother, Gillian, that her son would probably die. "That's what the doctor said to me. 'This is the most allergic kid I've ever seen.' He was telling me all these horror stories of kids who die at school. 'I don't know how you're going to make it through childhood,'" says Gillian, quoting him.

"He was horrendous. I was sobbing with my hivey, screaming baby," she says. "That was our introduction to the land of food allergies." She took the doctor at his word and figured they were doomed.

One day she was chatting with a friend whose son was as allergic as Jacob. The friend, Heidi Pasternak, mentioned that they were seeing a woman who was putting dairy on her son's skin, and he wasn't getting hives. Gillian knew that Heidi was constantly scanning scientific articles online, as she was, looking for breakthroughs in research, hunting for clinical trials her son might be eligible for, anything to give her hope. "I knew Heidi. She was by the book," says Gillian.

Heidi, of course, was the one whose word had had such a signifi-cant impact on Amanda Hanson, too. Heidi was like a bee, pollinating flowers.

Gillian called her parents. She called Jacob's pediatrician. She called a family friend who was an allergist. "All of them were like, 'I don't condone this. I definitely wouldn't use any food. But go see what the funny lady's doing.'" She felt like she'd gotten a little bit of permis-sion to give Amy's therapy a try.

Amy told Gillian that Jacob's anaphylactic incident with the for-mula was a traumatic event. She explained that Gillian herself had internalized all that fear and so had Jacob. "So I need you guys to deal with that, too," Amy told her. "Not just the food. I want you to take his brain over and tell him he can do it." Gillian completely got it.

The one thing that she had hammered into her son until that point was to be very afraid. And the lesson had sunk in. By the time he was five, the same year he started seeing Amy, he'd even stopped trusting his mother. "Mommy, did you wash your hands? Is that plate safe, Mommy?" he'd ask. "The older they are when they get to Amy, the more whacked they are by that stuff," Gillian says, meaning the harder it is to undo the paranoia.

Gillian grabbed hold of the mind-body component of the therapy and pushed ahead. Her husband pushed back. "Where's the proof? How can you tell him it's going to work?" Gillian's answer was, "I have to."

She understood that if the therapy was going to be successful, she needed Jacob to buy in, too. She started asking him about all the foods he wished he could eat. "It was such a weird reversal," she says now. They'd never talked about it before because it would have been too sad. "What do you see Mommy eat that you wish you could have?" she'd ask. He'd say, "I don't know what a doughnut tastes like."

Gillian started taking notes. The notes grew into songs as well as posters with pictures and promises. On one piece of poster board they drew three columns. In the first one, mother and son made a list of all the things he wanted to eat. The next column included a list of prizes he'd get once he overcame each allergy. Gillian told him, "Pick something I wouldn't normally give you." Jacob said, "Oh, like a toy gun?" Yes! "I would never buy you that," she said. "That's a great thing to write down."

The last column was about how he'd feel once he could eat the various foods again. He wrote, "I won't be scared when Mommy kisses me. She can't hurt me. I can go to school and not be scared."

Amy started encouraging all of her clients to make the same kind of poster. She called it a "vision board." As of this writing, Jacob, fourteen, has been eating everything for six years. Like Hayden Hanson and David Tsai, Heidi Pasternak's son, Lucas, is also still free of his allergies.

In the suburbs of Boston, word started to spread about what the funny lady was doing. Diane Lombardo heard about Amy on a field trip with her son, one of three, all of whom had severe allergies. Another mom mentioned that her previously anaphylactic son was now eating nuts. "I said, 'Give me her name.' I didn't think twice," Diane tells me.

A couple of weeks later Diane overheard two moms talking about Amy in the bleachers at a Little League game. "'Well, my daughter had dairy allergies and she's eating pizza!'" And there were murmurs in the line at school outside the nurse's office, among the parents who were dropping off their children's EpiPens in case they were needed. "What does she do? How does she do it?"

Diane called Amy and signed up her three boys. By then, the waiting list stretched to two years.

I first heard about Amy through word of mouth, too, from my sister, Rae, whose daughter, Indigo, has the fourteen food allergies. Or is it *had*? After being treated by Amy, Indigo now eats everything.

The next time Diane Lombardo took her kids in for their annual allergy checkup at Boston Children's, she asked the nurse if she'd heard of this lady Amy Thieringer. Diane had known the nurse since her oldest son was three months old and had his first allergic reaction. He was now twelve.

Yes, she had heard of her. "All I can tell you," the nurse said, according to Diane, "is that my patients who go see her don't come back to me."

"Don't they call you?" Diane asked.

"No. They're done," she said. And then she had a question for Diane. "When you go see her, can you tell me what she does?" (The nurse did not respond to messages seeking comment.)

By Amy's count, three hundred children have finished her program able to tolerate everything. They no longer need to see Amy, but they do need to keep eating the foods that had given them a problem. While it's impossible to verify that number independently, it's out of that group that I was able to confirm the sixty-five children whose parents say they are free of all of their allergies, including Diane Lombardo's three boys.

Almost to a person they described Amy to me as "life-changing." Diane says, "I pray for Amy every day."

Amy is careful to say that she's not curing allergies. Her therapy is a work-around. And she doesn't claim to be practicing medicine, either. She's an integrative nutrition and health coach.

Because her results are anecdotal, Amy and her collaborator, the BU psychologist and researcher Leslie Brody, had talked for a long time about doing a study to demonstrate the efficacy of Allergy Release Technique. "The treatment had been so helpful for me," Brody tells me, "and as a health researcher, I was very motivated to try to get it into the medical literature so that the treatment might be more widely disseminated." That way, researchers and clinicians could build on it, ultimately benefiting others as well as contributing to our understanding of allergies, she says.

So, after allergists at Boston Children's Hospital had arranged a meeting with Amy to hear about her therapy, Leslie Brody approached the group about collaborating on a study. Funding was raised from private sources, and the study moved ahead in early 2016. As of this writing, it is still under way.

❁   ❁   ❁

SCIENTISTS AT INSTITUTIONS ACROSS THE United States continue to plug away at a cure. There are a number of potential therapies, including herbal medicines, that are being looked at. Meanwhile, researchers are scaling back their expectations for oral immunotherapy because of the allergic reactions some children have had afterward. "I think everybody's looking at the fact that we're not going to cure this, at least with oral immunotherapy, the way we're going," says Dr. Hugh Sampson, the director of the Jaffe Food Allergy Institute and professor of pediatrics at the Icahn School of Medicine at Mount Sinai. "Our hope was that we would be able to cure people, to make them permanently tolerant, not that we still don't hope to do that, it's just that we realize it's a lot more complicated."

Dr. Sampson says that a more realistic goal is to use desensitization to give kids some defense against a severe reaction in case there is accidental exposure to the wrong food. "Maybe the most important thing is to protect people as opposed to being able to let them get out there and eat peanut butter sandwiches," he says. "We're dialing back our hopes."

I ask Dr. Sampson what he makes of the part of Amy's therapy that addresses anxiety. He's interested to hear about it. He tells me it reminds him of a study he read about when he was doing his fellowship, an allergy version of Pavlov's dog experiments.

Rats were sensitized to egg whites. Then one group of the animals was exposed to a flashing light and noise from a fan and injected with egg whites. As expected, the animals produced antibodies to the egg whites, as in the start of an allergic reaction. The group was put through this sequence—light and noise, egg whites, antibodies—over and over again.

Another group of sensitized rats got the same treatment but unpaired: they were injected a whole day after experiencing the light and noise.

Then both groups were injected with dummy egg whites while they were subjected to the light and noise. Nothing happened to the rats who'd experienced the light and noise separate from getting real egg whites before. But for the others whose injections were paired with the audiovisual cue before—bingo!—the light, noise, and injection of dummy egg whites were enough to produce an immune response.

And then there's that other phenomenon that's affiliated with the mind: the placebo effect. This is not to say that we can think our way out of allergies, but Amy's ultra-confidence that she can take care of a person's allergies is exactly the kind of manner and message that research has suggested is an important factor when people recover, whether they've received treatment or not. Or maybe the correct way to put it is that the assurance of the practitioner *is* the treatment in some cases.

The psychological aspect of Amy's therapy also reminds me of Harvard's Dr. Rediger and his ideas about how much sway our minds have. When Amy teaches an allergic child that he or she is now strong and safe and no longer vulnerable, it sounds like the mental change he's observed among people who've experienced spontaneous remission—realizing that they're not defective.

Science may one day shed more light on these mysteries. Frantic parents of allergic children, however, aren't willing to wait. Amy's wait list now stretches to four years.

One of those desperate, impatient parents is Dr. Ami Mehra, an internist with a subspecialty in allergy and immunology who practices in Chelmsford, Massachusetts. Her son, Ishaan, was so allergic to latex that he went into anaphylaxis after crossing paths with a clown whose balloon bounced off the boy's cheek. Dr. Mehra and her husband wondered how their son would ever be safe. He didn't have to play with balloons, but latex was everywhere. A lot of food is handled with latex gloves. So many kinds of produce were rubber-banded with latex. Tennis balls, pencil erasers. They sent Ishaan to school with his own special erasers, but what if other kids' erasers touched him?

"I was terrified, just terrified, scared out of my mind," Dr. Mehra says. "People would say to me, 'Wow, you're so lucky you're an allergist. At least you know what to do.' That would debilitate me because I was like, 'Yeah, what a joke I am. How limited I am. How unprepared I am to save this kid.'" She was a specialist in the exact disease her son had and there was nothing she could do for him. "I was losing hope and I was very aware of the limitations of medicine."

She was impressed with the results of desensitization in the literature, but she wasn't willing to try it on her own child. "I didn't have the experience. I wasn't prepared to treat my son as my first patient," she says.

In an attempt to further the science, she arranged a couple of dinners with venture capitalists and hedge fund managers. She told them, "Listen, you need to invest in food allergy research. This is a real problem." Dr. Mehra was honest with them. "It's affecting our children, and this is a really great way for you to get involved because you can make a deal and it would really help me."

Then she heard about Amy, the way everyone hears about Amy— from a friend. Dr. Mehra's friend happened to be an allergist at a top academic center. The doctor-friend said *she* had a friend whose child had been helped by Amy. She said that she'd also heard that Dr. Lynda Schneider, the director of the allergy program at Boston Children's, which would later undertake the study of Amy's therapy, knew about Amy. Dr. Mehra's friend encouraged her to find out more.

Dr. Mehra already knew Dr. Schneider and considered her a giant in the field. She sent her an email. Dr. Mehra says that Dr. Schneider's response was measured but that she didn't discourage her from seeing Amy. She explained, according to Dr. Mehra, that she could see why Amy's treating the anxiety component might be effective. For Dr. Mehra, the email was very important. (Dr. Schneider did not return calls seeking comment.)

Dr. Mehra called Amy. Amy told her that she could treat Ishaan's latex allergy. "I've never ever said that or heard that before, so of course that was attractive to me," Dr. Mehra tells me. Did part of her think it sounded crazy? "Of course!" she says. But she had nothing else. "I felt like we were definitely in uncharted waters and was very grateful for someone to throw me a life jacket. That's really what it felt like. I had a chance with Amy."

She didn't even worry that Amy's treatment might be putting her son at risk. "Knowing my child and how allergic he is," she says, "I felt that he was at risk with any type of desensitization." He was at risk just being in the world. Dr. Mehra was reassured by Amy's track record.

When Ishaan finally got in to see Amy, Dr. Mehra kept it from her allergist colleagues. As hopeful as she was about the process, she was afraid that the traditionally minded doctors she worked with would scoff at her.

After several months of seeing Amy, Ishaan went to a birthday party, walked through an arch of balloons, reached up, and felt them with his hands. And he was fine. At that point, Dr. Mehra came out of the closet to her fellow doctors.

The first thing they asked her was, "What is her number?"

Ishaan is now completely tolerant of latex. Dr. Mehra tells me that he even decided he wanted to chew on a balloon recently and put it in his mouth. All the same, she continues to write "latex allergic" on all of his forms. "Do I think it's permanent? I'm not sure!"

Amy has started training people in her therapy, including a pediatrician, nurses, nutritionists, and parents. She is excited that her protocol is being put to the test of science by Boston Children's—not because she cares about mainstream validation, but she would like to be able to reach more children. "If I can have a hospital as incredible as Children's validate it, then children's lives can start changing. Then hope can be given to this population," she says.

Her success has brought her enormous satisfaction. She's happy in her personal life, too. She's remarried and her three children, now grown, are regular visitors, callers, texters. Her son recently told her that it was her unconventional side that he loved most about her.

Gillian Epstein, who developed a close friendship with Amy over the course of her son Jacob's treatment, says that it's not confidence that makes Amy who she is. "Confidence implies that you know an outcome. 'Yes, I can do this. I've gotten a soccer goal before and I know I have it in me.' This is belief. Maybe it's more like religion or suspension of disbelief or something where you're really going out in the air in the middle of nowhere where you're saying, 'Okay, I'm somewhere I've never been,'" she says.

She compares Amy to a tightrope walker or someone who runs

across hot coals with bare feet. "They're doing insane crap. But they say, 'I can do this.' It's like, 'Really? Because it seems very dangerous.' But they can and they will," says Gillian.

"The track record is nothing. Each kid, having been a mom of one, is so dangerous. Every time it's crazy," says Gillian of her friend's work. "It's crazy brave."

14

Shepherd's Story, Part 3

The Surprise

Happy.
—Shepherd Meadows Strauss

One Saturday morning in 2015, Amy Thieringer pulled a pretzel from a silver tin, nicked off a poppy-seed-size speck with her fingernail, reached over to the pencil holder on her desk, selected a fork that she kept there along with a knife and spoon, and used it to place the shard of wheat on my son Shepherd's lower lip. On her command he reached his tongue out—showing himself to be a natural at lizarding—and pulled the glutinous scrap in.

Then he smiled.

Shepherd was seven. He'd been free of arthritis for three years. During that period, he'd been able to eat many things but still avoided gluten and dairy. The protein that lent wheat bread its squish had always been the most threatening one. We'd seen Shepherd, even after his initial recovery, feel pain within hours of accidental bites of the stuff. We believed that staying away from gluten was a major factor, if not the only factor, in controlling his arthritis.

Then we met Amy. After hearing about her from my sister, and seeing my niece, Indigo, overcome her allergies in Amy's care, I'd gone to Lexington, Massachusetts, to see if I could write about the therapy she'd developed.

When Amy agreed, and connected me to Amanda Hanson, she also suggested that she work with Shepherd. She said she could teach his body to tolerate gluten and dairy, just as she did for allergic kids like Hayden. She was taking a risk, letting someone write about her. She wanted to make sure that I really understood what she did. She would add a slot for him on Saturdays so that he wouldn't be jumping the list ahead of a child with a dangerous condition.

We paid the going rate, which at the time was $180 an hour. We drove up to Lexington every month from our home in Brooklyn, New York. Shepherd was five and a half when we started.

She had never worked with a child like Shepherd before, someone with JIA whose arthritis seemed to be triggered by certain foods. In typical Amy form, that didn't concern her. His body was making a mistake about certain foods, classifying them as enemies, she said, just like the allergic kids she saw. She knew how to work with that.

By then, Shepherd's diet wasn't as restricted as it had once been. He was eating nightshades again, that plant family that includes tomatoes and potatoes, and although his intake of sugar was still limited, he was allowed to indulge every so often and didn't have a problem when he did. He was down to keeping just gluten and dairy off-limits.

Amy would start with adding back in dairy. But first we needed to come up with a mantra for Shepherd to address any anxiety surrounding eating a forbidden food again. Amy recommended, "I'm healthy, strong, and powerful." She suggested talking to Shepherd about what superhero he wanted to be. This was how he'd picture himself while saying his mantra.

Shepherd said the Flash might be good because the wing-eared superhero was the fastest in the world and he—Shepherd—was fast, too. I said, "So maybe the mantra should be: 'I'm healthy, strong, and fast.'" His twin brother, Beau, who got in the act by picking Superman for himself, mentioned that the Flash could fly. Now *that* was good for the mantra. But then Darin got my attention and shook his head. He mouthed that in fact the Flash could not fly. Stickler. (Nerd.) So we were back to "healthy, strong, and fast."

Later, in the kitchen, out of the boys' earshot, Darin and I had a serious discussion about superpowers. Darin said that maybe the Flash was a bad choice because he was not that strong (no offense). But Shepherd was proud of his own speed and that represented his recovery. Plus speed required strength. Okay, we'd keep the Flash. The joys of being a neurotic parent.

The next morning, Shepherd decided to be Starscream, a Transformer. His new mantra, he said, was, "I'm very strong and I can fly in vehicle—no, plane—mode." A day later he was back to the Flash. He smiled when he said he was healthy, strong, and fast.

After a couple of months of groundwork laying in Amy's office, Shepherd ate a thin slice of a string cheese log. Within days, though, he began to seem stiff. He took the stairs in our house more slowly. When I gave him a little boost at the top one night, he said, "I love you." I told him that if he was feeling stiff he needed to remind the firefighters to take the day off, the firefighters being the well-meaning workers of his immune system that overreacted and caused damage even when they were trying to protect him. He said that he did that every day.

Amy said that Shepherd still had a real fear of dairy. She believed that that was causing his body to react the way he expected it to. Amy never expressed any doubt about what she thought was going on. I wondered if that had something to do with her lack of a medical background, that it liberated her from skepticism.

She reminded me of what happened with my niece Indigo and the pea. When Amy was working with her, it wasn't always a smooth process; it rarely is. One of Indigo's more stubborn allergies was to green peas. Every time my sister, Rae, would try to introduce a tiny piece of pea, Indigo would say her mouth felt funny. Finally, Amy suggested that Rae hide the pea in chocolate.

Sure enough, once the pea was in costume, Indigo didn't react to eating it. After several weeks of trickery, my sister revealed to Indigo that she'd been eating peas all along and didn't have a problem anymore. From that point on Indigo ate peas without issue. Rae had similar success when she hollowed out grapes and stuffed them with egg.

Shepherd had been on guard against dairy—and seen us fret about it—for almost half his life. When I told Shepherd that Amy said that he no longer had a sensitivity to dairy, he said, "How does she know?"

As much as I pretended otherwise, I was still fretting about all of this, too. Amy could tell and told me I needed to deal with my anxiety because Shepherd would pick up on it, and it would work against the process.

I'd probably always been a somewhat anxious person, but with the onset of Shepherd's arthritis, worries took over my mind in a bloodless coup. I got some relief when he recovered; I started sleeping better. But now that we were giving him the food we believed had played a role in his arthritis, I slid right back into my old what-if-ing.

Darin was out of town when Shepherd seemed to take a downturn after trying cheese again. He sent two emissaries in his place to help me through it. First my friend Margaret arrived on the scene with super heroic speed, her minivan as Batmobile. She brought me a lime tree. Then came my friend Phoebe, or, as I should call her, Robin.

I KEPT TRYING TO TALK to Shepherd about the firefighters. They were trying to protect him, which was causing the stiffness, but he didn't need them anymore because he was strong enough. He would say, "I don't want to talk about it, but I know." He'd cover my mouth with his hand. He'd been picturing himself as the Flash while he said his mantra and did his tapping—the vision and the words and the physical touch that could have a calming effect all serving as reminders that he wasn't vulnerable anymore. But now he replaced that powerful image with one of himself reading. Not an exact match to "healthy, strong, and fast."

The first day he was supposed to try ice cream again, we were on a trip to Paris. After dinner, we walked to a gelato place, but he wouldn't get anything. A five-year-old resisting ice cream. It tells you all you need to know about the power of fear. I finally talked him into trying a lick of mine. That was the breakthrough. And why wouldn't it be? What amount of apprehension can compete with caramel gelato?

The next day, Shepherd asked if he could get his own dish. He ordered caramel along with chocolate and pistachio. We were at that winning chain, Amorino, where they layer small slabs of gelato like rose petals.

That week, we talked Shepherd out of picturing himself reading while he said his mantra and I did his tapping, which I did every night, right after tucking him in. As much as he loved books, he seemed to have picked the image in an act of resistance to the program. Rather than pulling the Flash out of retirement as a replacement, he came up with something new: He would close his eyes and envision himself bouncing so high on the bed that he broke the roof and touched space. He stopped making funny faces while I tapped his face.

Sitting on the side of his bed, I lightly thumped the right points on his face and chest. One of them was under his arms, which we ended up cutting out of the routine because it tickled too much. Tapping the other points had the effect—every time—of making him yawn instantly.

Recently, I had to have surgery on my arm. When I came home from the hospital, Shepherd insisted on tucking me in and tapping my face. I can tell you, it felt wonderful.

Once Shepherd started taking the process seriously, his stiffness went away. Stiffness can also come and go, so it's impossible to say what made it fade in this instance.

We moved on to reintroducing gluten. Same deal. We started with one crumb of a pretzel, and he seemed stiff the next morning. Amy wasn't concerned. His body was "processing" the wheat, she said. Bumps were typical. We went up another crumb three days later.

Shepherd and I went out to our favorite spot for dinner, Prime Meats in Brooklyn. Darin and I split up the boys occasionally to spend one-on-one time with them, and also to let Beau get a real pizza fix. Shepherd and I both ordered pork chops, which we sent back when they arrived undercooked. While we waited, the waiter, bearded and apologetic, brought out a soft pretzel.

Shepherd was thrilled even though he couldn't eat it. He'd be able to eat it soon. He was already on his way. I suggested making crumbs from this pretzel for his daily ration. No, he wanted to save it. He confirmed with me that the entire thing was his, that he wouldn't have to share it once he was able to eat it. We agreed that it would be nice to get Beau his own. But Shepherd couldn't resist sharing some of it. He picked off the salt and ate it and wanted me to try it, too. He wanted me to smell how sweet the bread was and feel its warmth on my cheek. The pretzel was easy to grip, like a baby toy, a soundless bread rattle. Shepherd wouldn't let go of it. He didn't want to wrap it up. He didn't want it going in my purse. When we met back up with Beau and Darin, he held it behind his back to surprise them with it. He was eager that night to move up to three crumbs.

And yet, despite his comfort with the pretzel, the stiffness remained. It seemed like time to quit the whole endeavor. Before pulling the plug on gluten, though, Darin suggested we give deceit a try, à la Indigo and the pea. Amy was all for it.

So we told Shepherd that he was taking a break. He was going to go off wheat and dairy for a little while. We said this was Amy's suggestion, all part of her plan to make him even stronger. He didn't blink.

The first night I sliced open a bite of steak, inserted five pretzel bits, closed it back up like a surgeon, and stuck a fork in the top to hold it together, the tines like sutures. I added dairy milk to his almond milk. I had no idea what I'd say if he caught me. He seemed less stiff almost immediately.

We kept going. I buried the pretzel bits in frosting and gave him little spoonfuls. I tucked them under a blanket of dairy-free cheese on pizza. Gashes cut into sausages made good hiding places, too.

Then it was Halloween and the next day Shepherd took a downturn again. Darin and I had had to check the ingredient list on every piece of candy. We tried to be cool about it, but I'm sure Shepherd was aware of our worrying.

Enough already. We decided to stop trying to get Shepherd back on gluten. At the same time his rheumatologist, Dr. Kahn, noticed some slight stiffness at Shepherd's next checkup. After the exam, Darin took Shepherd out of the room so I could talk to Dr. Kahn privately. I told him that there was a possible explanation for the stiffness. We had reintroduced gluten, I said, cringing to admit it.

Dr. Kahn looked confused. His brow crinkled, but he kept listening. Then he said, "Clearly he has a sensitivity." Here was the guy who'd counseled us *not* to take anything out of Shepherd's diet, now pointing out to *me* that Shepherd had a problem with gluten. I was able to pick up on the irony despite the anxiety hives blooming along my jawline.

I assured Dr. Kahn that we were finished with gluten. Again, here I was assuring *him* that our food adventure was over. We didn't have the stomach for the knocks on the way to tolerance. And even if Shepherd would ultimately prevail, we couldn't run the risk of doing damage to his body. What a relief. I threw out the Prime Meats pretzel I'd been saving in the freezer.

We'd let him keep having dairy (out of the closet) since that one seemed to be okay. Getting one food group out of two back made a big difference in our lives. The cupcake options, for when he went to birthday parties, were much more delicious at the gluten-free bakery if you could tolerate dairy. If the price of keeping Shepherd healthy was eating crumbly, gluten-free bread, we had a deal. We'd already done it for years.

We were used to our gluten-free routine. We asked every waiter and waitress what was in the food. Then we asked if he or she was sure. We sent back gluten-free buns when they felt suspiciously un-cardboard-like to the touch, too soft, we thought, not to be wheat. Shepherd took his own food to parties, snacks on playdates, and pizza to school for Pizza Friday. Everyone else ate hot pizza from the Italian restaurant on the corner.

Even though all of this was old hat, we always, every time, felt bad for Shepherd. Not that he complained. And there seemed to be a constant influx of newer, tastier gluten-free options available, especially where we lived, in Brooklyn. But still, when I asked him how it felt not to be able to eat what everyone else was eating, he admitted that it bothered him. Of course it did. There is a huge social component to food, especially in a child's life.

The bigger concern was that if gluten remained the enemy, Shepherd would always be vulnerable to a flare-up. One bite away.

Which is how, nearly a year after we walked away from gluten, we found ourselves open to giving it another try. Shepherd had kept seeing Amy, and she'd continued to work on his tolerance of environmental allergens, which she said contributed to his overall reactivity.

Shepherd was better than ever. Over the years since he'd recovered there had been some issues unrelated to our food experiments. He had slightly sore wrists when the seasons changed one spring, which was solved after a short course of ibuprofen. When he went on long plane rides, he used to look a little stiff for a second after standing up. Sometimes in the morning, too. That never happened anymore and hadn't for a year.

One morning he told me his ankle hurt. I asked him if it felt like arthritis. He said he didn't remember what arthritis felt like. As I reveled in the beauty of those words, he said he'd twisted his ankle. Whatever it was was gone the same day.

We asked Shepherd if he wanted to try gluten again. In the past, he had said that he felt left out eating his own food. How would he feel if he could have gluten again? "Left in."

All right. One shot. The first sign of trouble and we would give up gluten for good.

Amy was wary of the risks of inflammation, too, but she was confident we could do this. We had to be all in, though. We would have to make posters and talk about all the stuff he'd be able to eat. Amy thought I seemed a lot less anxious about it than the time before and that that would make a difference. "I want him tapping. I want him saying his mantra," she said. This would remind him that he was strong and safe, taking his attention away from worrying.

Amy thought about how he could picture himself as he was saying his mantra. "I don't know if there's a superhero suit he can zip himself up in. I don't know if there's, like, shooting a goal in hockey, something that makes him feel empowered."

Shepherd ended up going with something a little more obvious: He imagined that his stuffed penguin, Pengie, was just born and weighed a hundred pounds. He would picture lifting him up, this arctic barbell, as a feat of strength. Okay. At other times he was a balloon inflating himself. My favorite nights were when he swam alongside his stuffed shark, holding one fin, while I got to hold the other. His mantra, which he came up with, was now, "I'm strong, healthy, happy, excited for Amy's, excited for everything."

He had one quibble. He didn't like the word "mantra." So instead I reminded him to say his "spiel." He asked, in all seriousness, if that was French for "mantra."

IT ALL ADDED UP TO that one crumb, that one smile, in Amy's office when he was seven. Crumbs don't usually see their names in lights. This one, though, was a really big deal. Just like before when we'd tried reintroducing gluten to Shepherd's diet, we added a single speck of a wheat product at a time. When that went so well, he started eating a couple more crumbs a day, then four, then twelve. We graduated to little measuring spoons, supplied by Amy, labeled "tad," "smidge," "dash," "pinch," and "drop," which I used to shovel more and more crushed pretzels into his mouth.

He worked his way up to sixteen pretzels in one go. Then Amy introduced crackers, then cookies, then bread.

SHEPHERD NOW EATS EVERYTHING. WE'RE making the rounds to all the eateries where he's been a spectator. So far, he's eaten a Vietnamese sandwich on the actual roll rather than dumping the chicken and vegetables onto a plate. The school carnival's coming up. After automatically checking the "no pizza" box on his permission slip, I had to send in a correction. We went back to Prime Meats for a pretzel. I asked him how he felt about eating it. "Happy," he said.

Now that I know how critical dietary fiber is to maintaining gut bacteria health, I do feel a little conflicted about this cascade of refined flour. When Shepherd ate his first Oreo at school, the smallest voice in my head asked, *What have you done?* He was thrilled, however. He'd drawn a picture of one on his "vision board" six months before.

Once Shepherd finishes his victory lap, I plan on zeroing in on whole grains for the family except for special occasions. He needs to eat wheat every day to hold his tolerance, Amy says. *The Good Gut* by Justin and Erica Sonnenburg is a good guide. Chapter 5 is called "Trillions of Mouths to Feed." Justin Sonnenburg makes his own bread from flour he grinds himself to preserve more of the wheat's fiber. Is this what it's going to take to look out for Shepherd and Beau's little bacteria friends?

Shepherd did not have a single moment of stiffness or pain during the six-month reintroduction process. Afterward, when the seasons changed, his wrist was briefly, slightly sore again, but a sonogram showed no inflammation.

As with all of these stories, I'll say it again: It's impossible to draw conclusions from a single result. But given what we now know about how the composition of our microbiome can shape a healthy immune response or be related to disease, it seems to me that it's a strong possibility that Shepherd's illness and recovery were rooted in his gut, as Dr. Fasano speculated.

Shepherd's tolerance to gluten could also stem from restoring his gut bacteria. Just as an unhealthy microbiome can bring on intolerance, so, too, can a reinvigorated population make the food issues go away, says Jamie Stelter's Dr. Lipman, who sees it in his practice.

I also believe that if Amy hadn't helped Shepherd get over his fear of eating gluten and dairy, he would have continued to react to those foods. I think of those mice that had an immune response to nothing but a shot of fake egg whites and a little commotion. Amy's therapy may be working on a gut level, too—stress can impact our microbiota, according to a 2015 review in *Frontiers in Psychiatry*.

And then, of course, there's Amy's attitude: the fearless conviction that she can do it, the exact bearing that science tells us can bring about healing. Amy says that children are much easier to treat than adults. Maybe it's because they simply believe her. They haven't learned yet to doubt what they can't understand. For a lot of us who've been through Amy's process, one of the biggest challenges was being told we had to believe that it would work because if we didn't, it wouldn't.

It's also possible that gluten never was the problem for Shepherd. If he can tolerate it now, maybe he could tolerate it before, too, and we just misinterpreted events, even though he repeatedly had flare-ups after eating gluten. Then again, Amy's machine showed that he was extremely sensitive to gluten when she first tested him. After months of working with Amy, he tested normal. But it's still hard to know what to make of the machine.

Shepherd continues to take fish oil and probiotics, but he's been able to stay off methotrexate. He doesn't complain when his mother dumps Swiss chard and chia seeds in smoothies for him—and for his microbes. He remains taller than his identical twin, Beau, which he never fails to rub in. His behind, which he's been known to wiggle, now fills out the seat of his pants. He swims, scoots, has a nice backhand.

I no longer get hives on the days Shepherd has a checkup with the rheumatologist. I actually looked forward to a recent visit, excited to tell Dr. Kahn that Shepherd seemed healthier than ever to me. "What do you attribute that to?" he asked me.

At that recent visit, Dr. Kahn tested every one of Shepherd's joints, as he always did. I noticed that when he checked Shepherd's fingers, he held his hand the way you do when you propose to someone. When Dr. Kahn was through, he had one word: "Wow."

With Shepherd feeling so good, I finally had the courage to ask a question I'd been afraid to ask for four years. What were the odds that the arthritis would come back? Because even though we thought we knew why he'd gotten better, we didn't actually know anything. Dr. Kahn's face fell ever so slightly and only for a second. "It's a good question," he said, quickly resuming his usual upbeat tenor. He said that no one really knew because there weren't good long-term studies of kids with JIA. And since Shepherd's case was so unusual—kids like him weren't supposed to go off medication—there was even less information.

Okay, but should we, at least, feel encouraged by this long stretch of good health? Dr. Kahn gave the kind answer. Of course we should, he said.

I can still remember the night years ago after Dr. Kahn had examined Shepherd and found for the first time that he had no active arthritis. Shepherd was four and still slept in his little toddler bed. I kissed him good night and told him to give me five. "For the no arthritis?" he asked. I nodded, holding out my hand. He slapped my palm again and again, over and over. It sounded like clapping.

Afterword

The Landing

FIVE YEARS AGO I STEPPED OUT ONTO THE FRONTIER OF MEDICAL science, first as a parent, then as a journalist. I did not think I'd end up here. I tried things I never imagined I'd try, to help Shepherd have a decent life.

I started working on this book a year after Shepherd had wowed us with his startling recovery from arthritis. I was not expecting a second act—that he would one day eat gluten and dairy again. Before I met Amy Thieringer I never thought that it might be possible.

Annie Salafsky and Jamie Stelter surprised me, too. When I first spoke to them, I was drawn to the never-give-up spirit they shared— the theme of this book. Annie was also floundering on her mission to stop Tess's insistent seizures, and Jamie was handicapped by a bad limp.

Although I wasn't aiming to represent the entire range of possible results when you try anything and everything, I did want to present a mixed picture. I was wary of overpromising what poorly understood approaches to health could do. This is another reason I decided to tell Annie's and Jamie's stories—*because* they hadn't triumphed.

And then the stories took over, and I had to follow. Shepherd rocketed over his last hurdle. Annie's doggedness paid off when they finally discovered the likely source of her daughter's seizures. And although Jamie has had to endure multiple surgeries since I met her, we get to leave her while she's "walking like a total boss."

But what are we to make of these stories, of all of the recoveries in this book? Because stories are anecdotes, and anecdotal evidence does not demonstrate cause and effect—proof that a therapy works. So we don't know why the people in these pages got better or whether their recoveries will stick. And we can't say if other people will benefit from the courses they followed.

But these stories do suggest potential targets for new research, which *will* bring answers. Some of this research, as I've reported, is already under way.

Other meanings are more concrete. In Annie's case, the value of what she ultimately was able to do for Tess is clear: find the right doctor, Dr. James Owens, who thought to look again, when others hadn't, for what might be causing Tess's seizures and discovered the tumor. If Annie had accepted her daughter's fate, if she hadn't been so relentless, Tess may have lost her chance to overcome her seizures.

Annie's story is a good reminder that even if a person feels she's tapped out of conventional medicine—that science has nothing left to offer her—she might want to take a third, fourth, fifth look. Not giving up means not closing yourself off to the most knowledgeable people. Even Jamie, who ventured into the unknown, still came home to traditional medicine for the kind of fix it does especially well: surgically repairing her ankle.

I'D GONE INTO THIS PROJECT thinking that these people, these stories, might offer hints about the human body and disease. What I also realized was how little we know. The experience has been like learning a foreign language. Only when you start to get better at speaking it can you fully appreciate what fluency is—and how far you are from it. Much further than you thought you were when you said your first *bonjour.*

One of the more disheartening surprises of researching this book was learning that some of what we think we know may not be that solid after all. Our vast body of biomedical literature may be distorted by industry money. Financial relationships among pharmaceutical companies, scientific investigators, and academic institutions are widespread, and the conflicts of interest arising from these ties can influence the science, according to a 2003 review in *JAMA.* When industry funds studies, the benefits of their drugs and other products are often exaggerated while potential harms are downplayed, write the authors of a 2013 review in the *European Journal of Clinical Investigation.* They concluded that the tentacles of industry are so entangled with healthcare that the practice of medicine itself is biased. "In many medical fields, as much as ninety percent of the published information that doctors rely on is flawed," says Dr. John Ioannidis, a professor of medicine at the Stanford University School of Medicine and a director of the Meta-Research Innovation Center at Stanford.

The profit motive also has a heavy hand in setting the American research agenda. In 1980, the drug industry funded only a third of all biomedical research. By 2000, that number had nearly doubled to 62 percent, according to the *JAMA* review. So, to a large degree, we're deciding what to research based on whether a potential therapy can be patented and profited from.

I USED TO DISMISS THE weird and the out-there. That way I ran no risk of looking dumb or gullible.

Now, even some doctors, including ours, are starting to say things like: If it works, I don't have to understand it. Most of us recognize that science is always evolving, and there is still so much we don't know about illness. Given that, who's to say that any possible solution is out of the question? Things that we can't explain now may become the paradigm of tomorrow.

Researchers, especially, know that a discovery can come from anywhere, but they need funding to be able to look. At the back of the book, I've included a list of scientists and organizations I consulted in writing this book, along with information about their work. One thing everyone seems to agree on: We need to know more.

OVER THE LAST FIVE YEARS our understanding of the microbiome and its connection to our health has grown. It's pretty clear at this point that one of the most important things we can do for our bacteria has been right in front of us the whole time, on our dinner plates.

The explanation is simple. To keep a diverse, plentiful population of bacteria thriving, you have to feed it. And you have to feed it food that will make it all the way to the large intestine where the bacteria live. Refined, processed foods are digested before they can get that far along in our gastrointestinal tract. So our trashy American diet is basically starving our helpers. It's a mass die-off, exacerbated by the use of antibiotics and bacteria-killing hand-sanitizers, as Justin and Erica Sonnenburg write in *The Good Gut*. When our bacteria disappear, they can't do their job of calibrating our immune system properly, among other critical tasks.

But. *But.* The fiber in whole fruits, vegetables, grains, legumes, seeds, and nuts is tough enough to survive the trip to the colon. So when we eat foods rich in fiber, we're also providing nourishment to our bacteria in the gut. And when a wide variety of bacteria species thrives, they help protect us from disease. "Based on everything we know about the microbiota, eating lots of dietary fiber is probably the single best way we can improve the state of our gut!!" Erica Sonnenburg writes to me in an email. The double exclamation points are hers. But the enthusiasm is mine, too.

She and her husband argue that we shouldn't wait for proof. "Scientists are trained to be highly skeptical," they write in their book. "So it is not in our nature to provide recommendations unless they have been put through the rigors of a double-blind, placebo-controlled study." And yet, they say there is enough scientific evidence so far, some of which they've produced in their own lab at Stanford, to begin to make diet and lifestyle adjustments to optimize the health of the microbiota. These microbiologists feel confident saying that feeding our microbes "is one of the most important choices we can make for our health."

"We know that the typical American diet is not healthy," says Erica Sonnenburg, "and that a high-fiber diet reduces the risk of all-cause mortality. Whether a high-fiber diet is providing its benefit through the microbiota is still not definitively established, but a lot of arrows are pointing in that direction. I think it is prudent at this point to assume that improving the state of one's microbiota through diet will be beneficial to the maintenance of one's health."

The upshot of decades of scientific inquiry may very well turn out to be: Eat your vegetables. "They're good for you," says your mom.

Talking about healthy food makes our friend Dr. Fasano happy. "Okay," he says. "Now you bring me to where I want to be. If I feed junk food to a mouse, this mouse will develop colon cancer. I can make this fellow very sick. That really speaks volumes. Many of these conditions are due to our attitude toward nutrition. Again, I see, how to say, circumstantial evidence—not definite proof, because we don't have the tools yet—but circumstantial evidence that this is what's going on here."

Some of us can't wait until all the evidence is in.

EARLY ON, I WASN'T HOPEFUL that we'd find a way out of Shepherd's illness. I didn't go looking to experiment. But now, if someone in my family got sick with an impossible illness, I'd know to get to work. I've learned that I'm not helpless—that we aren't. We have some control and an enormous amount of choice in terms of what kinds of therapies to pursue.

So I'd make a long list of doctors, and it won't surprise you to know I wouldn't stop there. After all, what the people in this book show is that perseverance, taking control, can work.

If I need to be more positive, I'll think of Jamie. If I need to question the premise, I'll think of Annie. If I need courage, I'll think of everyone.

YOU HAVE TO FIGURE IT out on your own. It was Ashton Embry, a father *and* a believer in science, who told me that. Before his charity funded Terry Wahls's research, he was the one who decided on *his* own that a Paleo diet might help his son's MS, and his symptoms did improve. "Thank God for the Internet," Embry tells me. "That's made all the difference, getting across the information and the people. I'm a scientist. Nothing is for certain. You always question, question, and question."

Do we run the risk of fooling ourselves? We have a lot to learn yet about the power of the mind. But based on what we know already, that a belief in recovery can sometimes help us get there, I wonder if there is even such a thing as false hope.

The other day, Shepherd, now eight, saw *The Adventures of Tintin*, the movie based on the Hergé comics. He said that the story had a moral I would like. At one point, the Captain Haddock character says, "You hit a wall, you push through it." Shepherd seemed to realize then that the idea sounded familiar. "Like me!" he said. "With arthritis!" He raised his palms, shoved them forward like a bulldozer, and said: "Push!"

Acknowledgments

The thing I learned about books, writing one for the first time, is that there wouldn't be any without the generosity of others.

To Terry, Amanda, Jamie, Annie, Amy Chan, and Amy Thieringer. Thank you for trusting me with your stories. You answered a thousand questions—sometimes tedious, often painful—with uncommon grace, and an eye toward helping people. I guess I shouldn't be surprised that you didn't quit on me, but I am so grateful nonetheless.

To my friend first and agent second, Bill Clegg, the one who, more than anyone, made this book happen, starting with slapping the table and telling me I had to do it. Writing the book was just a fancy excuse to talk to you more often.

To Kate Medina. Your ability to turn a manuscript into a book is a wonder. Thank you for that, but also, and perhaps just as crucial, all the x's and o's along the way.

To the many doctors, scientists, and other experts who gave their time and lent me their knowledge, even reading over passages to make sure I got things right. Your participation and effort were invaluable, and not only to my ability to sleep. Thank you so much.

To Char Walker. Thank you doesn't quite cut it. See: Changed life, Shepherd.

To my early readers. Darin Strauss, Phoebe Lichty, Rae Meadows, Ronny Meadows, Jessica Reaves, Sabrina Felson, and Jeff Giles. What a coup that my friends and family members also happen to be excellent writers and/or doctors or nursing students. Your suggestions were critical and your encouragement was everything.

To Taylor Beck. Thank you for everything you taught me (which was a lot), for all your enthusiasm (more than a lot), and for every last neuron diagram you drew for me on café napkins (I've lost count).

Thank you also to Dr. Phil Kahn, a walking testament to how much a doctor's kindness matters.

To Joel Lovell, Catherine Barnett, and Margaret Cordi for sharing your gift for words.

To Fred Guterl and Henry Rabinowitz. There's no appreciation like the appreciation for someone who keeps you from looking dumb, or at least tries to.

To the Random House team: Erica Gonzalez, Anna Pitoniak, Barbara Fillon, Mary Moates, Christine Mykityshyn Theresa Zoro, Leigh Marchant, Andrea DeWerd, Benjamin Dreyer, Thomas Perry, Ted Allen, Amelia Zalcman, Paolo Pepe, Joseph Perez, Susan Turner, Toby Ernst, Carolyn Foley, and Gina Centrello. What an absolute honor and pleasure to work with all of you.

In the category of love, support, and willingness to listen even though you must have gotten very sick of hearing about the book, I'd like to nominate: Tom Watson, Katie Goldstein, Marc Sternberg, Michael Handelman, Lewis Krauskopf, Andrea Truncali, Celene Ryan, Amanda Robb, Lisa Miller, Kira Smith, and, last and most, the Meadows family: Jane, Ron, Ronny, and Rae. My first stroke of luck was becoming one of you. Mom, you were the original rule-challenger. Your example has sure served me well.

Speaking of luck, to the Strausses and Hechlers: I love you guys.

To Shepherd and Beau, what it's all for. Madly, madlier, madliest.

And to Darin. I don't know how other people who don't have you do it. I love you.

Diary of a Gut

———

Terry Wahls's Menu on August 26, 2016

MORNING

A smoothie:

3 cups leaves: lemon balm, dandelion leaves and root (all gathered
    fresh from the garden)

1 tbsp lemon juice

2 tbsp flaxseed

⅓ 13.5 fl. oz. can coconut milk

4–5 cups water

One chicken leg left over from the night before

NOON

She skips lunch.

EVENING

Another smoothie:

3–4 cups parsley, mint, rosemary, savory, and chicory leaves (again,
    fresh from the garden)

1 tbsp lime juice

2 tbsp green banana flour

⅓ 13.5 fl. oz. can coconut milk

4–5 cups water

Lamb chops marinated in rosemary and lemon juice, grilled

Red bell pepper, yellow bell pepper, and portabella mushrooms, grilled

Cauliflower "rice": cauliflower minced in a food processor and sautéed with fresh oregano, basil, and savory from the garden; coconut oil; and ghee.

One whole head of garlic, grilled ("This is delicious!" Terry says), which is expressed and mixed into the cauliflower.

Chia pudding: coconut milk, chia seeds, and nutmeg—no sweetener. Topped with five large blackberries.

Chamomile tea and coconut milk

⅓ can coconut milk to top the meal

The Evidence for Omega-3s and Probiotics

There's reason to believe that some of the other interventions we tried—beyond diet—may have been beneficial for Shepherd, too. Omega-3 fatty acids may be "modestly helpful" in relieving symptoms of rheumatoid arthritis in adults, according to the National Institutes of Health's National Center for Complementary and Integrative Health.

The effect of omega-3s on children with inflammatory arthritis has been studied less, but the existing science is encouraging. In a randomized, double-blind, placebo-controlled trial published in *World Journal of Pharmaceutical Research* in 2015, sixty-six children with JIA were divided into two groups. One group got 2,000 milligrams of omega-3s a day; the other got a placebo. After twelve weeks, the mean number of joints affected by arthritis dropped significantly among the thirty children in the omega-3 group who completed the study, as did levels of inflammatory markers in their blood, compared to the kids who took a placebo. In a 2012 *Clinical Rheumatology* study that looked at similar measures, almost 100 percent of the children with JIA who were given omega-3s—twenty-five out of twenty-seven—improved after twelve weeks.

Of course, these are only two small trials, the second of which lacked a placebo, but the results are strikingly positive. Even though fish oil is stuck in the dissed alternative medicine category, it's hard to believe that there is not broader interest in outcomes like that. "I think that all the time," UCSF's Dr. Newmark tells me. "I wonder, 'Didn't anybody see this study?'"

WHAT DO OMEGA-3S DO? WHEN we eat them, they get incorporated into the walls of immune cells in the blood. From there, they inhibit the production of a certain enzyme that leads to inflammation, scientists at UCSD reported in 2012 in *Proceedings of the National Academy of Sciences of the United States of America.*

This anti-inflammatory function may have therapeutic implications way beyond arthritis to a broad range of diseases that involve inflammation, including cancer, obesity, diabetes, and heart disease.

Omega-3s have so far shown some benefit in people with depression, ADHD (attention deficit hyperactivity disorder), schizophrenia, and mild cognitive impairment, according to a 2016 review in the *Journal of Nutrition & Intermediary Metabolism,* although evidence is still emerging and there's controversy in the literature. When heart disease patients took omega-3s, their risk of death decreased, one meta-analysis indicated, but some trials have been disappointing.

Dietary omega-3s have also been reported to protect the cells that line the intestinal wall from "pro-inflammatory insults"—great term—"and accelerate recovery from inflammation." This may reduce intestinal permeability, write the authors of the 2016 review.

Researchers say that probiotics hold enormous potential for restoring a healthy population of gut bacteria, but so far the evidence is thin. A couple of different strains have been shown to reduce joint inflammation in mice, says Dr. Fergus Shanahan, the chairman of the department of medicine at University College, Cork, in Ireland, and the director of the APC Microbiome Institute. He makes the point that probiotics are not a monolith; each strain is different. "In the same way that not all pills are the same. Probiotics are live microorganisms and differ from one another hugely. No one would suggest that a pill which helps arthritis would also help high blood pressure."

In a 2012 meta-analysis in *PLoS ONE* of studies involving 10,351 patients, eleven different species of probiotics were found to have a positive effect on eight gastrointestinal diseases. One primary way probiotics work, the authors write, is by reducing increased gut permeability.

The Sonnenburgs write in *The Good Gut* that there is growing evidence that probiotics, which they describe as "transient visitors to the gut," can help reduce our chance of getting certain infections. "People who consume probiotics are better able to fight off colds, flu, and diarrheal illness." But which strains of bacteria? I ask Erica Sonnenburg. "Because each person has a somewhat unique microbiota and a unique genetic makeup, it is difficult to point to a specific strain of probiotic as being beneficial for a certain infection," she says. Until scientists are able to "type" our microbiotas and provide specific probiotic recommendations, we can try to find strains that work best with our system through trial and error, on an individual basis, she says. But it's also a numbers game—"just getting a lot of probiotic bacteria in your system to try to rev up your immune system."

Because, like all supplements, probiotics can bypass government safety and efficacy standards, the Sonnenburgs suggest getting extra beneficial bacteria by eating fermented foods rather than gamble on a pill. Yogurt, kefir—a dairy drink—and sauerkraut all supply probiotics. Dr. Fergus Shanahan, the Irish probiotics expert, has advice, too. "The best way the public can select a probiotic is to purchase only from a reputable supplier with high quality-control standards and with clinical and experimental supporting data," he says. In Shepherd's case, we opted for the rare probiotic that requires a prescription—VSL#3—so we could be confident about what it was.

Bang for Your Broccoli

The Best Sources of Fiber, Omega-3 Fatty Acids, and Antioxidants

Fiber bars and supplements aren't an alternative to eating well. When it comes to getting valuable nutrients, "you cannot beat food," says Kristin Kirkpatrick, manager of wellness nutrition services at the Cleveland Clinic Wellness Institute. She shows us where to look for the central players in this book.

Fiber

- Cruciferous vegetables: cauliflower, broccoli, brussels sprouts. "Those are huge," Kirkpatrick says.
- Berries. A half cup of raspberries, for example, has 8 grams of fiber, which puts you well on your way to the minimum 35 grams a day that Kirkpatrick recommends for men and women.
- Don't peel that apple! Fruit skins are a great source of fiber.
- Whole grains. But stick to the purest form. "I will only recommend intact grains, instead of a whole grain bread or pasta because they had to be processed," says Kirkpatrick. And the more processed something is, the less nutrient-dense, the less fiber it has. "Yeah, whole wheat is better than white," she says, "but I'd rather someone go with quinoa, wheat berries, oats, brown rice, buckwheat."
- Instead of whole grain pasta, try one that's bean-based. It's about "upgrading your carbs," says Kirkpatrick. Pasta made from beans

will provide 12 grams of fiber and you also get many antioxidants, she says. "Go beyond what you've been told." Even in the case of oats. "What kind of oatmeal? Is it quick-cooked? We can make that better."

- Dried fruits—dates, apricots, prunes—have a lot of fiber because they're so concentrated. But don't have a lot of these, Kirkpatrick says, because they can be high in sugar, even if it's not added, and sugar is highly inflammatory.

Omega-3 Fatty Acids

- Omega-3s come in two versions: the marine form, from seafood, and plant-based. Marine omega-3s, called EPA (eicosapentaenoic acid) and DHA (docosahexaenoic acid), are the kinds of fatty acids we need. The omega-3s in plants—ALA (alpha-linolenic acid)— have to be converted by our bodies into EPA and DHA. Some of the nutrients are lost in the process, so marine is a superior source, says Kirkpatrick.
- Salmon is the best place to get omega-3s, and wild is better than farmed. The omega-3s are higher quality because the fish are getting them from algae and other sea vegetables, Kirkpatrick says. Canned salmon is always wild, she points out. Frozen salmon is another option for saving money.
- Other good sources: wild lake trout, sardines, cod liver oil, halibut. Eating a fatty fish two to three times a week gets you to the minimum recommendation.
- Of the plant-based options, walnuts are excellent because they offer fiber and antioxidants, too. "See how many qualities you can get in one food," says Kirkpatrick.
- Hemp seeds are rich in omega-3s and protein: "It kills two healthy birds with one stone."
- Flaxseeds. High in fiber, but unless you grind them, you won't access the omega-3s.
- Chia seeds offer fiber and omega-3s, too. No pulverizing required.
- Soy, but make sure it's in its whole form, like edamame.

- Tuna has omega-3s, but it's also high in mercury, so consumption should be limited.
- In the omega-3 supplement world, quality is key, says Kirkpatrick. "You don't want a farmed fish that's processed," she says. "You want to know where your omega-3 oil is coming from." Quality pretty much dictates price. What about krill oil? "We don't know as much about it," she says.

Antioxidants

"Think of it simply as color," says Kirkpatrick. "The color that is provided to plants often will signify the amount of antioxidants involved, and the deeper the hue, the better the benefit." So, she recommends getting at least five colors of fruits and vegetables a day.

Some examples:

- Yellow: pineapple and bell peppers
- Purple/Blue: black beans, blackberries, blueberries, purple carrots
- Red: strawberries, tomatoes, apples, cherries, red onions, red wine, raspberries, cranberries, beets
- Orange: turmeric, pumpkin, sweet potatoes
- Green: watercress, spinach, avocado, brussels sprouts, broccoli, kale, green tea, matcha tea
- White/Brown: walnuts, whole grains, mushrooms, coconut, cauliflower, cocoa, black and white tea

Keep in mind that cooking changes the chemical compositions of vegetables, which influences the concentration and availability of their nutrients. Whether there's a positive or negative effect seems to vary according to the vegetable and the cooking method, though the data are not complete. Better to steam or boil carrots, zucchini, and broccoli, rather than fry them, for example. But any kind of cooking increases the antioxidants in these three vegetables, according to a study in the *Journal of Agricultural and Food Chemistry*.

The Work Left to Be Done

—

BECAUSE THESE STORIES OF RECOVERY ARE ANECDOTAL, SCIENtific study is needed to understand what they might mean for others. Here are the names of some of the experts and groups I consulted in the writing of this book, in order of appearance, who are working toward finding answers. You can find more information about them and their research at the websites listed below. Keep in mind that website addresses can change.

Dr. Jeffrey Rediger: medicineofhopeandpossibility.com

Dr. Alessio Fasano: celiaccenter.org

Veena Taneja: mayoclinic.org

Justin and Erica Sonnenburg: sonnenburglab.stanford.edu

Dr. Terry Wahls: terrywahls.com/about/the-wahls-foundation

DIRECT-MS, Ashton Embry's research and educational organization: direct-ms.org

The National MS Society: nationalmssociety.org

Amy Thieringer: allergyart.com. The Allergy Release Technique pilot study: bostonchildrens.org/ARTStudy

Leslie Brody: bu.edu

Dr. Alexander Khoruts: microbiota-therapeutics.umn.edu. For people wanting more information about FMT research, Dr. Khoruts suggests: achievingcurestogether.org

Dr. Fergus Shanahan: apc.ucc.ie

Dr. M. Flint Beal: brainandmind.weill.cornell.edu/beal-laboratory

Dr. Hugh Sampson: icahn.mssm.edu/research/jaffe

Dr. Wesley Burks: med.unc.edu/pediatrics/specialties/air/food-allergy

Angela Duckworth: angeladuckworth.com

Autism Speaks: autismspeaks.org

Dr. Corinne Keet: hopkinsmedicine.org/johns-hopkins-childrens-center

Dr. Orrin Devinsky: faces.med.nyu.edu

Kristin Kirkpatrick: my.clevelandclinic.org/services/wellness

The Documenting Hope Project. While not discussed in this book, this group's interests align with issues raised here. Its study's aim is to understand how chronic illnesses in children develop and what treatment strategies may be most effective for recovery. Documenting hope.com

Glossary

allergen: Any substance that causes an allergic reaction.

allergic reaction: When the immune system mistakenly registers a harmless substance, such as a peanut or tree pollen, as dangerous and launches a response that can include hives, nasal congestion, and difficulty breathing (anaphylaxis).

alternative medicine: Therapies developed outside of and used in place of mainstream medicine.

anaphylaxis: A life-threatening allergic reaction that can cause the airways to close.

antibodies: Proteins produced by the immune system to fight off substances that are identified as a threat.

antigen: Any substance that elicits an immune response, specifically the production of antibodies against it.

antioxidants: Abundant in fruits and vegetables, antioxidants are vitamins or other substances that can protect against cellular damage.

attention deficit/hyperactivity disorder (ADHD): Often diagnosed in children, typical behavior includes hyperactivity, impulsivity, and difficulty paying attention.

autism: A developmental disorder characterized by social difficulties, problems with communication, and repetitive behaviors. Also called autism spectrum disorder.

autoimmune disease: A disorder in which the body's immune system mistakenly attacks healthy tissues.

casein: A protein in milk.

celiac disease: An immune response to eating gluten that can damage the small intestine, affecting the proper absorption of nutrients.

Clostridium difficile (C. diff): A kind of bacterium that can cause severe diarrhea, infections of which have been successfully treated with FMT.

cognitive behavioral therapy (CBT): A form of psychotherapy that teaches a person to examine stressful events critically and notice exaggerated thoughts, so as not to get swept up in them.

complementary medicine: Therapies developed outside mainstream medicine used in conjunction with it. Also called integrative medicine.

DNA: A molecule in our cells that carries genetic instructions.

electroencephalogram (EEG): A test that measures electrical activity in the brain.

elimination diet: Cutting out many foods at once, such as dairy, wheat, corn, soy, eggs, nuts, and citrus, then adding them back in one at a time to see how the body responds.

epilepsy: A neurological disorder characterized by unpredictable seizures.

epinephrine: A lifesaving drug that works in part by relaxing the muscles in the airways of a person experiencing anaphylaxis. It comes prefilled in EpiPens, an automatic injecting device.

fecal microbiota transplantation (FMT): The transferring of stool from a healthy donor to the intestine of someone else for therapeutic purposes, usually via colonoscopy.

fiber: The part of a plant that remains after the small intestine has digested all it can.

functional medicine: A healthcare approach that aims to find the underlying causes of chronic disease rather than just treat the symptoms.

gluten: The name for the proteins in wheat, rye, and barley.

increased intestinal permeability: A condition in which the normally tight junctions between the cells of the intestinal wall loosen, potentially allowing harmful bacteria or other materials into the tissues. Also referred to as "leaky gut."

inflammation: The heat, swelling, redness, and pain that are the immune system's weapons against infection and damaged tissue.

integrative medicine: Therapies developed outside mainstream medicine used in conjunction with it. Also called complementary medicine.

juvenile idiopathic arthritis (JIA): An autoimmune disease that involves painful and damaging inflammation in the joints of children.

leaky gut: A condition in which the normally tight junctions between the cells of the intestinal wall loosen, potentially allowing harmful bacteria or other materials into the tissues. Also called "increased intestinal permeability."

legumes: The family of plants that includes peanuts, beans, and peas.

microbiome: The collective genetic material of the microbes—mostly bacteria—that live in or on the human body. The term is often used to refer to the community of microorganisms itself.

microbiota: The community of microbes—mostly bacteria—that lives in and on the human body.

mitochondria: The units within most of our cells that convert fuel into energy, among other tasks.

multiple sclerosis (MS): Considered by most experts to be an autoimmune disease, it can disrupt the brain's ability to communicate with the body's muscles.

National Institutes of Health (NIH): Part of the U.S. Department of Health and Human Services and comprised of twenty-seven institutes and centers, it's the country's medical research agency, supporting scientific study.

naturopathic medicine: Emphasizing stress reduction, nutrition, and herbal supplements, among other interventions, it combines healing practices developed hundreds of years ago with more modern primary care.

nightshades: A family of plants that includes potatoes, tomatoes, peppers, and eggplant.

omega-3 fatty acids: A type of fat molecule, found in salmon and other fatty fish, that is essential to certain functions in the body and may reduce inflammation.

Paleo diet: Modeled after the diet early humans are thought to have had, it emphasizes meats, eggs, fruits, and vegetables and doesn't allow dairy, grains, refined sugar, or legumes.

Parkinson's disease: A progressive neurological disorder that affects movement and coordination.

placebo effect: The healing that occurs when you believe a treatment will make you better.

polyarticular JIA: Inflammatory arthritis in children that affects five or more joints.

post-traumatic stress disorder (PTSD): The persistent reliving of a shocking or dangerous experience after it's over.

probiotics: Supplements of bacteria that are either the same or similar to the microorganisms found naturally in the body.

rheumatoid arthritis (RA): As opposed to the wear and tear that causes osteoarthritis, RA is the result of a malfunctioning immune system, which attacks the joints, causing painful swelling and destruction.

secondary progressive MS: A stage of the disease, often following a less severe form, marked by a steady worsening of neurological function and disability.

seizure: Abnormal activity in the brain—too many neurons firing at once—that can lead to injury, brain damage, and sudden death.

Specific Carbohydrate Diet: No grains, no starches, no added sugar, no milk. It's intended to restore balance to gut bacteria.

spontaneous remission: When a disease vanishes on its own for reasons we don't understand.

zonulin: A protein that increases the permeability of the intestinal wall.

Selected Bibliography

1 **Shepherd's Story, Part 1: *The Leap***

Offit, Paul, MD. *Do You Believe in Magic? The Sense and Nonsense of Alternative Medicine.* New York: HarperCollins (2013).

3 **Shepherd's Story, Part 2: *The Science of Our Guts***

Horton, Daniel B., et al. "Antibiotic exposure and juvenile idiopathic arthritis: a case-control study." *Pediatrics* 136(2) (2015).

Hvatum, M., et al. "The gut-joint axis: cross reactive food antibodies in rheumatoid arthritis." *Gut* 55(9): 1240–1247 (2006).

Meadows, Susannah. "The Boy with a Thorn in His Joints." *The New York Times Magazine,* February 3, 2013.

Offit, Paul A., MD. *Do You Believe in Magic? The Sense and Nonsense of Alternative Medicine.* New York: HarperCollins (2013).

Sender, Ron, Shai Fuchs, and Ron Milo. "Revised estimates of the number of human and bacteria cells in the body." *PLoS Biology* 14(8): e1002533 (2016).

Sonnenburg, Justin and Erica Sonnenburg, PhDs. *The Good Gut: Taking Control of Your Weight, Your Mood, and Your Long-Term Health.* New York: Penguin Press (2015).

4 **Terry Wahls:** *How Far Can Moxie Take You?*

Beal, M. Flint. "Bioenergetic approaches for neuroprotection in Parkinson's disease." *Annals of Neurology* 53(s3): S39–S48 (2003).

Bourre, Jean-Marie. "Effects of nutrients (in food) on the structure and function of the nervous system: update on dietary requirements for brain. Part 1: micronutrients." *The Journal of Nutrition, Health & Aging* 10(5): 377–385 (2006).

Bourre, Jean-Marie. "Effects of nutrients (in food) on the structure and function of the nervous system: update on dietary requirements for brain. Part 2: macronutrients." *The Journal of Nutrition, Health & Aging* 10(5): 386–399 (2006).

Lemon, Jennifer A., Douglas R. Boreham, and C. David Rollo. "A complex dietary supplement extends longevity of mice." *The Journals of Gerontology: Series A* 60(3): 275–279 (2005).

McPherron, Shannon P., et al. "Evidence for stone-tool-assisted consumption of animal tissues before 3.39 million years ago at Dikika, Ethiopia." *Nature* 46(7308): 857–860 (2010).

Offit, Paul, MD. *Do You Believe in Magic? The Sense and Nonsense of Alternative Medicine.* New York: HarperCollins (2013).

Wahls, Zach with Bruce Littlefield. *My Two Moms: Lessons of Love, Strength, and What Makes a Family.* New York: Gotham (2012).

Warinner, Christina (2013). "Debunking the Paleo Diet": Christina Warinner at TEDxOU [video file]. Retrieved from http://tedxtalks .ted.com/video/Debunking-the-Paleo-Diet-Christ.

5 **Diet and Inflammation:** *Terry Looks for Proof*

Bisht, Babita, Terry L. Wahls, et al. "Multimodal intervention improves fatigue and quality of life in subjects with progressive multiple sclerosis: a pilot study." *Degenerative Neurological and Neuromuscular Disease* 2015(5): 19–35 (2015).

Bisht, Babita, Terry L. Wahls, et al. "A multimodal intervention for patients with secondary progressive multiple sclerosis: feasibility and effect on fatigue." *Journal of Alternative and Complementary Medicine* 20(5): 347–355 (2014).

Reese, David, Terry L. Wahls, et al. "Neuromuscular electrical stimulation and dietary interventions to reduce oxidative stress in a secondary progressive multiple sclerosis patient leads to marked gains in function: a case report." *Cases Journal* 2: 7601 (2009).

Wahls, Terry L. (2011). "Minding Your Mitochondria." TEDxIowaCity [video file]. Retrieved from: https://www.youtube.com /watch?v=KLjgBLwH3Wc.

Wahls, Terry, MD with Eve Adamson. *The Wahls Protocol: How I Beat Progressive MS Using Paleo Principles and Functional Medicine.* New York: Avery (2014).

6 The Science of Success: *What Makes Us Try and Try Again*

Duckworth, Angela. *Grit: The Power of Passion and Perseverance.* New York: Scribner (2016).

Duckworth, Angela (2013). "Grit: The Power of Passion and Perseverance." TED talk [video file]. Retrieved from: https://www.ted .com/talks/angela_lee_duckworth_grit_the_power_of_passion_and _perseverance.

7 Amanda Hanson: *Love and Sacrifice*

Dhond, Rupali P., Norman Kettner, and Vitaly Napadow. "Do the neural correlates of acupuncture and placebo effects differ?" *Pain* 128 (1–2): 8–12 (2007).

Feinstein, David, PhD. "Acupoint stimulation in treating psychological disorders: evidence of efficacy." *Review of General Psychology* 16: 364–380 (2012).

Furillo, Andy. "Family Sues City After Girl's Peanut-Allergy Death at Camp Sacramento." *The Sacramento Bee,* April 18, 2014.

Keet, Corinne A., et al. "Long-term follow-up of oral immuno-therapy for cow's milk allergy." *The Journal of Allergy and Clinical Immunology* 132(3): 737–739 (2013).

Keet, Corinne A. and Robert A. Wood. "Emerging therapies for food allergy." *The Journal of Clinical Investigation* 124(5): 1880–1886 (2014).

Napadow, Vitaly, et al. "Effects of electroacupuncture versus manual acupuncture on the human brain as measured by fMRI." *Human Brain Mapping* 24(3): 193–205 (2005).

Napadow, Vitaly, et al. "The status and future of acupuncture mech-anism research." *The Journal of Alternative and Complementary Medicine* 14(7): 861–869 (2008).

Sicherer, Scott H., et al. "US prevalence of self-reported peanut, tree nut, and sesame allergy: 11-year follow-up." *The Journal of Allergy and Clinical Immunology* 125(6): 1322–1326 (2010).

8 Jamie Stelter: *The Raw Fuel of Optimism*

De Filippis, Francesca, et al. "High-level adherence to a Mediter-ranean diet beneficially impacts the gut microbiota and associated metabolome." *Gut* 65(11): 1812–1821 (2016).

Dyche, Lawrence and Deborah Swiderski. "The effect of physician solicitation approaches on ability to identify patient concerns." *Journal of General Internal Medicine* 20(3): 267–270 (2005).

Hagen, Kåre Birger, et al. "Dietary interventions for rheumatoid arthritis (Review)." *Cochrane Database of Systematic Reviews* (1): 1–53 (2009).

Haghikia, Aiden, et al. "Dietary fatty acids directly impact central nervous system autoimmunity via the small intestine." *Immunity* 43(4): 817–829 (2015).

Kaptchuk, Ted J., et al. "Components of placebo effect: randomized controlled trial in patients with irritable bowel syndrome." *The BMJ* 336(7651): 999–1003 (2008).

Kjeldsen-Kragh, J., et al. "Controlled trial of fasting and one-year vegetarian diet in rheumatoid arthritis." *The Lancet* 338(8772): 899–902 (1991).

Mullen, Seamus. *Seamus Mullen's Hero Food.* Kansas City: Andrews McMeel Publishing (2012).

The Physicians Foundation. 2014 Survey of America's Physicians. http://www.physiciansfoundation.org/uploads/default/2014 _Physicians_Foundation_Biennial_Physician_Survey_Report.pdf.

Sköldstam, L., L. Hagfors, and G. Johansson. "An experimental study of a Mediterranean diet intervention for patients with rheumatoid arthritis." *Annals of Rheumatoid Diseases* 62(3): 208–214 (2003).

Sonnenburg, Justin and Erica Sonnenburg, PhDs. *The Good Gut: Taking Control of Your Weight, Your Mood, and Your Long-Term Health.* New York: Penguin Press (2015).

9 **The Science of the Mind and Body: *"Things Shift Toward Wellness"***

Amanzio, Martina and Fabrizio Benedetti. "Neuropharmacological dissection of placebo analgesia: expectation-activated opioid systems versus conditioning-activated specific subsystems." *The Journal of Neuroscience* 19(1): 484–494 (1999).

Benedetti, Fabrizio. "Placebo and the new physiology of the doctor-patient relationship." *Physiological Reviews* 93(3): 1207–1246 (2013).

Benedetti, Fabrizio, Antonella Pollo, and Luana Colloca. "Opioid-mediated placebo responses boost pain endurance and physical performance: is it doping in sport competitions?" *The Journal of Neuroscience* 27(44): 11934–11939 (2007).

Benedetti, Fabrizio, et al. "Placebo-responsive Parkinson patients show decreased activity in single neurons of subthalamic nucleus." *Nature Neuroscience* 7(6): 587–588 (2004).

Goebel, Marion U., et al. "Behavioral conditioning of immunosuppression is possible in humans." *The Faseb Journal* 16(14): 1869–1873 (2002).

Mayo Clinic. "Placebo effect: enhancing healing." Mayo Clinic Health Letter (April 2014).

McRae, Cynthia, et al. "Effects of perceived treatment on quality of life and medical outcomes in a double-blind placebo surgery trial." *Archives of General Psychiatry* 61(4): 412–420 (2004).

Meissner, Karin, et al. "The placebo effect: advances from different methodological approaches." *The Journal of Neuroscience* 31(45): 16117–16124 (2011).

Petrovic, Predrag, et al. "Placebo in emotional processing–induced expectations of anxiety relief activate a generalized modulatory network." *Neuron* 46(6): 957–969 (2005).

10 Annie Salafsky: *Saying No to No*

Devinsky, Orrin, et al. "Cannabidiol in patients with treatment-resistant epilepsy: an open-label intervention trial." *The Lancet Neurology* 15(3): 270–278 (2016).

Hsiao, Elaine Y., et al. "Microbiota modulate behavioral and physiological abnormalities associated with neurodevelopmental disorders." *Cell* 155(7): 1451–1463 (2013).

Reardon, Sara. "Bacterium can reverse autism-like behaviour in mice." *Nature: News* (December 5, 2013).

Zlokovic, Berislav V. "The blood-brain barrier in health and chronic neurodegenerative disorders." *Neuron* 57(2): 178–201 (2008).

11 The Science of Hope: *Agency vs. Learned Helplessness*

Christanson, John P., Steven F. Maier, et al. "Anxiogenic effects of brief swim stress are sensitive to stress history." *Progress in Neuro-Psychopharmacology and Biological Psychiatry* 44: 17–22 (2013).

Hammack, Sayamwong E., Steven F. Maier, et al. "Corticotropin releasing hormone type 2 receptors in the dorsal raphe nucleus mediate the behavioral consequences of uncontrollable stress." *The Journal of Neuroscience* 23(3): 1019–1025 (2003).

Ryan, Bryce C. and John G. Vandenbergh. "Intrauterine position effects." *Neuroscience & Biobehavioral Reviews* 26(6): 665–678 (2002).

Seligman, Martin E. P. and Steven F. Maier. "Failure to escape traumatic shock." *Journal of Experimental Psychology* 74(1): 1–9 (1967).

Seligman, Martin E. P., Steven F. Maier, and James H. Geer. "Alleviation of learned helplessness in the dog." *Journal of Abnormal Psychology* 73(3): 256–262 (1968).

12 Trusting Her Son: *Amy and Jaxon Chan Take On ADHD with Diet*

Campbell, Eric G., et al. "Physician professionalism and changes in physician-industry relationships from 2004 to 2009." *Archives of Internal Medicine* 170(20): 1820–1826 (2010).

Carter, C. M., et al. "Effects of a few food diet in attention deficit disorder." *Archives of Disease in Childhood* 69(5): 564–568 (1993).

Chowdhury, Rajiv, et al. "Association of dietary, circulating, and supplement fatty acids with coronary risk: a systematic review and meta-analysis." *Annals of Internal Medicine* 160(6): 398–406 (2014).

Dana, Jason and George Loewenstein. "A social science perspective on gifts to physicians from industry." *JAMA* 290(2): 252–255 (2003).

Egger, J., et al. "Controlled trial of oligoantigenic treatment in the hyperkinetic syndrome." *The Lancet* 325(8428): 540–545 (1985).

Fasano, Alessio, MD with Susie Flaherty. *Gluten Freedom: The Nation's Leading Expert Offers the Essential Guide to a Healthy, Gluten-Free Lifestyle.* New York: Wiley (2014).

Kupferschmidt, Kai. "Scientists fix errors in controversial paper about saturated fats." *Science* (March 24, 2014).

Millichap, J. Gordon and Michelle M. Yee. "The diet factor in attention-deficit/hyperactivity disorder." *Pediatrics* 129(2): 1–8 (2012).

Morrow, Richard L., et al. "Influence of relative age on diagnosis and treatment of attention-deficit/hyperactivity disorder in children." *Canadian Medical Association Journal* 184(7): 755–762 (2012).

Newmark, Sanford, MD. *ADHD Without Drugs: A Guide to the Natural Care of Children with ADHD.* Tucson: Nurtured Heart Publications (2010).

Pelsser, Lidy M., et al. "Effects of a restricted elimination diet on the behaviour of children with attention-deficit hyperactivity disorder (INCA study): a randomised controlled trial." *The Lancet* 377(9764): 494–503 (2011).

Sonnenburg, Justin and Erica Sonnenburg, PhDs. *The Good Gut: Taking Control of Your Weight, Your Mood, and Your Long-Term Health.* New York: Penguin Press (2015).

13 Amy Thieringer: *Evolution of a Healer*

Brody, Leslie R., et al. "Coping strategies, life themes, and HIV nondisclosure in autobiographical narratives in relation to HIV viral load and HAART adherence in women with HIV." Paper presented at the American Public Health Association, Chicago (November 2015).

Brody, Leslie R., et al. "Gender role behaviors of high affiliation and low self-silencing predict better adherence to antiretroviral therapy in women with HIV." *AIDS Patient Care and STDs* 28(9): 459–461 (2014).

Brody, Leslie R., et al. "Life lessons from women with HIV: mutuality, self-awareness, and self-efficacy." *AIDS Patient Care and STDs* 30(6): 261–273 (2016).

Gamlin, Linda. "Mast cells respond to Pavlovian conditioning." *New Scientist* (January 28, 1989).

Long, Tom. "Max Coffman, 95; Delivery Boy Became Store Tycoon." *The Boston Globe*, July 1, 2005.

MacQueen, G., et al. "Pavlovlian conditioning of rat mucosal mast cells to secrete rat mast cell protease II." *Science* 243 (4887): 83–85 (1989).

14 Shepherd's Story, Part 3: *The Surprise*

Gur, Tamar L., Brett L. Worly, and Michael T. Bailey. "Stress and the commensal microbiota: importance in parturition and infant neurodevelopment." *Frontiers in Psychiatry* (February 2015).

Afterword: *The Landing*

Bekelman, Justin E., Yan Li, and Cary P. Gross. "Scope and impact of financial conflicts of interest in biomedical research: a systematic review." *JAMA* 289(4): 454–456 (2003).

Sonnenburg, Justin and Erica Sonnenburg, PhDs. *The Good Gut: Taking Control of Your Weight, Your Mood, and Your Long-Term Health.* New York: Penguin Press (2015).

Stamatakis, Emmanuel, Richard Weiler, and John P. A. Ioannidis. "Undue industry influences that distort healthcare research, strategy, expenditure and practice: a review." *European Journal of Clinical Investigation* 43(5): 1–7 (2013).

The Evidence for Omega-3s and Probiotics

Abou El-Soud, N. H., et al. "A randomized double-blind placebo-controlled trial of omega-3 supplementation in juvenile idiopathic arthritis: improvement in disease activity and functional status." *World Journal of Pharmaceutical Research* 4(8): 2764–2772 (2015).

Gheita, Tamer, et al. "Omega-3 fatty acids in juvenile idiopathic arthritis: effect on cytokines (IL-1 and TNF-α), disease activity and response criteria." *Clinical Rheumatology* 31(2): 363–366 (2012).

Lee, Lai Kuan, et al. "Docosahexaenoic acid-concentrated fish oil supplementation in subjects with mild cognitive impairment (MCI): a 12-month randomised, double-blind, placebo-controlled trial." *Psychopharmacology* 225(3): 605–612 (2013).

Milte, C. M., et al. "Increased erythrocyte eicosapentaenoic acid and docosahexaenoic acid are associated with improved attention and behavior in children with ADHD in a randomized controlled three-way crossover trial." *Journal of Attention Disorders* 19(11): 954–964 (2015).

Norris, Paul C. and Edward A. Dennis. "Omega-3 fatty acids cause dramatic changes in TLR4 and purinergic eicosanoid signaling." *Proceedings of the National Academy of Sciences of the United States of America* 109(22): 8517–8522 (2012).

Pawelczyk, Tomasz, et al. "A randomized controlled study of the efficacy of six-month supplementation with concentrated fish oil rich in omega-3 polyunsaturated fatty acids in first episode schizophrenia." *Journal of Psychiatric Research* 73: 34–44 (2016).

Peet, Malcolm, et al. "Two double-blind placebo-controlled pilot studies of eicosapentaenoic acid in the treatment of schizophrenia." *Schizophrenia Research* 49(3): 243–251 (2001).

Phillips, Michelle A., et al. "No effect of omega-3 fatty acid supplementation on cognition and mood in individuals with cognitive impairment and probable Alzheimer's disease: a randomised controlled trial." *International Journal of Molecular Sciences* 16(10): 24600–24613 (2015).

Radcliffe, J. E., et al. "Controversies in omega-3 efficacy and novel concepts for application." *Journal of Nutrition & Intermediary Metabolism* 5: 11–22 (2016).

Rapaport, Mark Hyman, et al. "Inflammation as a predictive biomarker for response to omega-3 fatty acids in major depressive disorder: a proof-of-concept study." *Molecular Psychiatry* 21(1): 71–79 (2016).

Ritchie, Marina L. and Tamara N. Romanuk. "A meta-analysis of probiotic efficacy for gastrointestinal diseases." *PLoS ONE* 7(4) (2012).

Sonnenburg, Justin and Erica Sonnenburg, PhDs. *The Good Gut: Taking Control of Your Weight, Your Mood, and Your Long-Term Health.* New York: Penguin Press (2015).

Sperling, Lawrence and John R. Nelson. "History and future of omega-3 fatty acids in cardiovascular disease." *Current Medical Research and Opinion* 32(2): 301–311 (2016).

Wen, Y. T., J. H. Dai, and Q. Gao. "Effects of omega-3 fatty acid on major cardiovascular events and mortality in patients with coronary heart disease: a meta-analysis of randomized controlled trials." *Nutrition, Metabolism, and Cardiovascular Diseases* 24(5): 470–475 (2014).

Willemsen, Linette E. L., et al. "Polyunsaturated fatty acids support epithelial barrier integrity and reduce IL-4 mediated permeability in vitro." *European Journal of Nutrition* 47(4): 183–191 (2008).

Bang for Your Broccoli: *The Best Sources of Fiber, Omega-3 Fatty Acids, and Antioxidants*

Miglio, Christina, et al. "Effects of different cooking methods on nutritional and physicochemical characteristics of selected vegetables." *Journal of Agricultural and Food Chemistry* 56(1): 139–147 (2008).

Index

About the Author

SUSANNAH MEADOWS is a former senior writer for *Newsweek*. She has been a frequent contributor to *The New York Times*, most recently writing a column for the Arts section about books along with reviews. The stories she's covered include the 2004 presidential campaign, the aftermath of 9/11, Columbine, Hurricane Katrina, and the Duke lacrosse scandal. She has appeared on *CBS This Morning, CNN, MSNBC, Fox News, ESPN, Charlie Rose,* and *The Brian Lehrer Show.* She lives with her husband and twin sons in Brooklyn.

susannahmeadows.com

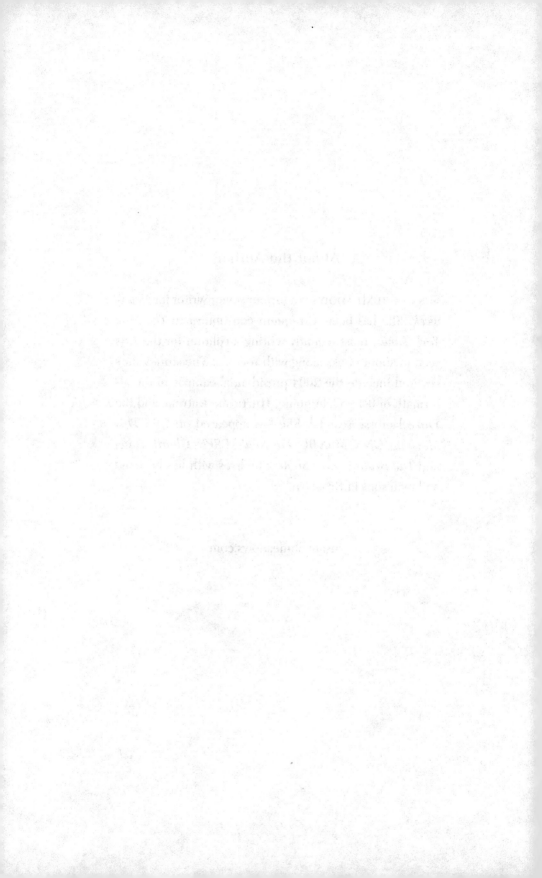

About the Type

This book was set in Caledonia, a typeface designed in 1939 by W. A. Dwiggins (1880–1956) for the Merganthaler Linotype Company. Its name is the ancient Roman term for Scotland, because the face was intended to have a Scottish-Roman flavor. Caledonia is considered to be a well-proportioned, businesslike face with little contrast between its thick and thin lines.